APPLIED EPIGENETICS
FOR MENTAL HEALTH PROFESSIONALS

APPLIED EPIGENETICS
FOR MENTAL HEALTH PROFESSIONALS

Onoriode Edeh, M.D.
Kyle J. Rutledge, D.O., Ph.D.

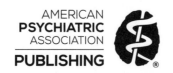

AMERICAN
PSYCHIATRIC
ASSOCIATION
PUBLISHING

Copyright © 2024 American Psychiatric Association Publishing

ALL RIGHTS RESERVED

First Edition

Manufactured in the United States of America on acid-free paper

27 26 25 24 23   5 4 3 2 1

American Psychiatric Association Publishing
800 Maine Avenue SW, Suite 900
Washington, DC 20024–2812
www.appi.org

Library of Congress Cataloging-in-Publication Data

Names: Edeh, Onoriode, author, editor. | Rutledge, Kyle J., author, editor.
    | American Psychiatric Association Publishing, publisher.
Title: Applied epigenetics for mental health professionals /
    authors/editors, Onoriode Edeh, Kyle J. Rutledge.
Description: Washington, D.C. : American Psychiatric Association
    Publishing, [2024] | Includes bibliographical references and index.
Identifiers: LCCN 2023036161 (print) | LCCN 2023036162 (ebook) | ISBN
    9781615374137 (paperback : alk. paper) | ISBN 9781615374144 (ebook)
Subjects: MESH: Mental Disorders--genetics | Epigenesis, Genetic
Classification: LCC RC455.4.G4 (print) | LCC RC455.4.G4 (ebook) | NLM WM
    140 | DDC 616.89/042--dc23/eng/20230831
LC record available at https://lccn.loc.gov/2023036161
LC ebook record available at https://lccn.loc.gov/2023036162

British Library Cataloguing in Publication Data

A CIP record is available from the British Library.

Contents

Contributors

Kai Anderson, M.D.
Associate Director, Psychiatry Residency; Assistant Professor of Psychiatry; Director of Psychotherapy Training; Director of Ambulatory Behavioral Health Services, Central Michigan University College of Medicine, CMU Medical Education Partners, Saginaw, Michigan

Onoriode Edeh, M.D.
Clinical Assistant Professor of Psychiatry, Central Michigan University College of Medicine, CMU Medical Education Partners, Saginaw, Michigan

Caroline Gobran, M.D.
Resident Physician, Beaumont Psychiatry Residency, Beaumont Health, Dearborn, Michigan

Haley Rutledge, M.S.
Previously, University of California Davis School of Medicine, Department of Medical Microbiology and Immunology, Davis, California

Kyle J. Rutledge, D.O., Ph.D.
Clinical Assistant Professor of Psychiatry, Central Michigan University College of Medicine, CMU Medical Education Partners, Saginaw, Michigan

Disclosures

The following contributors stated that they had no competing interests during the year preceding manuscript submission:

Kai Anderson, M.D.; Onoriode Edeh, M.D.; Caroline Gobran, M.D.; Haley Rutledge, M.S.; Kyle J. Rutledge, D.O., Ph.D.

Preface

Epigenetics is growing. As geneticists and biologists extend our knowledge of the cellular concepts and molecular phenomena that affect gene expression without changing the gene sequence, the science is expanding into other areas. Developmental trajectories, environmental effects on gene expression, and inherited phenotypes rely heavily on epigenetic mechanisms. The field of medicine has found novel applications of epigenetics in better understanding how pathology develops and the potential for characterizing—and in some cases producing—novel treatments.

The field of psychiatry is no exception. The study of epigenetics has grafted itself onto this branch of medicine, fostering new perspectives for understanding neurodevelopment across the life span, including neurodevelopmental and neurodegenerative disorders, family dynamics and shared environments, effects of trauma and life stressors, resilience, mood disorders, and the influence of lifestyle factors on healthy aging. The recognized impact of epigenetics is also represented in questions on in-training, licensing, and board exams. As it adds to our understanding of how pathology arises, epigenetics also provides fresh perspectives on interventions that may revitalize hope for providing relief to patients seeking our help.

That being said, the rate of growth of epigenetics in the field of psychiatry is outpacing the average psychiatric practitioner's level of familiarity with the topic. To understand the applications of epigenetics to our field, practicing psychiatrists, nurse practitioners, physician assistants, psychologists, trainees, and students increasingly encounter clinical research that is remarkably complex, encompassing epigenetic mechanisms and pathways that are outside the scope of their preclinical training.

This book is a resource to the behavioral health or psychiatric practitioner who is interested in keeping up with the field of applied epigenetics within psychiatry. The first chapter, "Overview of Genetic and Epigenetic Mechanisms," provides a refresher on genetic mechanisms necessary to grasp the core concepts and machinery of epigenetics. The chapter is by no means comprehensive, as it is intended for an audience that has previously completed coursework in genetics and molecular biology, but it includes a concise review of all the major concepts that arise in current applications of epigenetics in psychiatry. Much more detailed information is available in outside sources, but the content presented here is discussed at a level which, if mastered, will provide a sufficient understanding for the reader to dive with confidence into new literature on the topic.

The next chapters provide overviews of how epigenetics has improved our understanding of specific clinical aspects in psychiatry: mood disorders with a focus on depression (Chapter 2, "Epigenetic Modulation in Major Depressive Disorder"); neurological disorders (Chapter 3, "Epigenetics in Neurodevelopmental and Neurodegenerative Disorders"); trauma, toxic stress, and resilience (Chapter 4, "Epigenetics of Childhood Trauma and Resilience"); and health-promoting behaviors (Chapter 5, "Epigenetics of Lifestyle and Aging"). The goal for this book is not for readers to become experts in epigenetics in psychiatry, but rather for physicians and providers to fill the gaps in their knowledge of the core science of epigenetics enough to confidently approach and comfortably grasp current and future research in pathology and treatment of psychiatric disorders.

A note about language.   We recognize the expansive and nonbinary nature of human gender expression. In this book, without yet having a clear alternative, we use traditional binary terms such as *male/female* and *maternal/paternal*, but we support proposals for more inclusive language.

Acknowledgments

Turning an idea into a book is an experience that is both internally challenging and rewarding. I especially want to thank the individuals who provided support in various capacities in making a reality out of this book. To my wife (Samantha Edeh), thank you for always being there for me and for always supporting my dreams. Your frequent reminders and encouragements are unparalleled and kept the motivation during the entire process. I want to give honor to my alma mater, the University of Ibadan, Nigeria, for a well-grounded educational support and for nurturing my interest in science and fostering positive values. THANK YOU. The world of medicine is a better place thanks to mentors who take the time to share the gift of knowledge with future doctors. Special thanks to Dr. John Covault and Dr. Debra Forrest of the University of Connecticut; Dr. Molly Wimbiscus and Dr. Tatiana Falcone of the Cleveland Clinic; and Dr. Asif Khan of Central Michigan University College of Medicine, who provided encouragement and insight through this process.

Onoriode Edeh, M.D.

To the kind-hearted Dr. Harold B. Lenhart, empathic psychiatrist, curious philosopher, wise teacher, and inspirational human being. A big thank-you to Haley Rutledge, M.S., for being my personal genetics/epigenetics tutor throughout medical school, producing images for this book, correcting our early drafts, being my wife and putting up with me, and most importantly, for giving our children—Sydney, Harvey, and Josephine—healthy genes AND a great environment. Keeping with the theme, an additional hearty thank-you to my own mom and dad (others call them Cathy and Paul) for the genes and the healthy environment they tirelessly provided, and finally to my brother, Jeremy, for always keeping my developmental trajectory on a positive (but never-too-serious) track, present time included.

Kyle Rutledge, D.O., Ph.D.

Overview of Genetic and Epigenetic Mechanisms

Onoriode Edeh, M.D.
Haley Rutledge, M.S.
Kyle J. Rutledge, D.O., Ph.D.

To understand epigenetics, it is crucial to first grasp the central concepts of genetics. As noted in the Preface, this first chapter is meant to provide a consolidated overview of genetic mechanisms relevant to epigenetic functions. The enzymatic reactions and lasting chemical marks of **epigenetics** cannot occur outside the context of genetics. To comprehend why epigenetics affects traits of an individual, one must first understand what genes are and how they are expressed in the first place. Therefore, in this chapter we present a concise review of the major concepts of genetics, presented side by side with the high-yield principles of epigenetics, to form a stable base for understanding the specific applications of epigenetics in psychiatry in the chapters that follow.

DNA Structure

Deoxyribonucleic acid (DNA) is essential to life. DNA contains heritable, functional units known as **genes**. Genes are sequences of nucleotides within the DNA that act as instructions for the creation of functional molecules. Traditionally, genes encode proteins, but many also encode noncoding **ribonucleic acid (RNA)** as the final functional molecule. The length of each gene varies depending on the size of the protein or RNA that it encodes. The human genome describes all the genetic information in the cell contained by 23 **chromosomes**. Each chromosome contains hundreds to thousands of genes and millions of DNA base pairs.

DNA consists of two chains of **polynucleotides**, each link consisting of a **nucleotide** made of three components: a **nitrogenous base** (base), a **pentose sugar**, and a phosphate group (see Figure 1–1). Bases include purine bases—guanine (G) or adenine (A)—or pyrimidine bases—cytosine (C), thymine (T), or uracil (U). Nucleotides forming DNA use **deoxyribose** as the pentose sugar and G, A, C, or T as the bases; RNA nucleotides use **ribose** as the pentose sugar with bases G, A, C, or U. The base is covalently bonded to the pentose sugar, and the pentose sugar is esterified to the phosphate group. Nucleotides are connected to each other by a phosphodiester bond in such a way that the phosphate group forms the backbone and confers a negative charge to the polynucleotide. The bases are usually oriented to face the medial position and form hydrogen bonds when paired, stabilizing the DNA double helix.

An important detail to note in the nucleotide is that the phosphate (negatively charged) group is attached to the carbon in the 5′ (pronounced "five prime") position, and a hydroxyl group is attached to the carbon in the 3′ position of the cyclic pentose sugar. This creates a directionality, or polarity, of the strand that guides transcriptional machinery and is relevant for naming conventions. The double-stranded polynucleotides of DNA are oriented in opposite directions, referred to as **antiparallel**.

A **nucleoside** comprises only a base and a pentose sugar (i.e., a nucleotide without a phosphate group). Adenosine is perhaps the most familiar nucleoside, owing to its medical application in treating heart arrhythmia and its relevance in adenosine triphosphate (ATP). Other nucleosides include guanosine, thymidine, cytidine, and uridine.

The entirety of genetic information usually expressed in the form of various observable traits (or **phenotypes**) and nonobservable traits is stored in the DNA inside the nucleus of the cell. DNA cannot leave the nucleus of the cell; therefore, another temporary molecule (RNA) is used to carry the exact DNA sequence out of the nucleus into the body of the cell where the protein-making machinery resides. This process of converting genetic information, or the **base sequence**, of the DNA into RNA is termed **transcription**. **Messenger RNA (mRNA)** moves outside the nucleus and is translated from nucleic acid sequences into amino acid se-

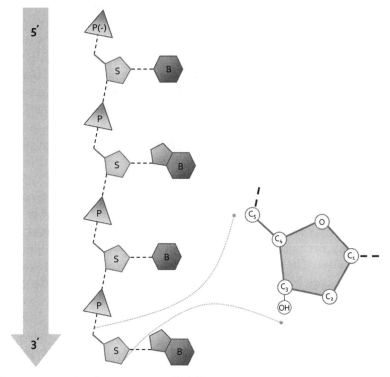

Figure 1–1. Basic structure of DNA.

Simplified version of a tetranucleotide, depicting the interaction between the various components in the DNA. A nucleotide comprises a nitrogenous base (B), a pentose sugar (S), and a phosphate unit (P). The bases typically orient medially when forming a double helix. The phosphate group provides a negative charge and is bonded (esterified) to the sugar via a phosphodiester bond, forming the backbone of the DNA. Within the pentose sugar, carbon atoms are numbered C_1 through C_5 based on position. Note the polarity of the strand, following a 5′-to-3′ directionality, named based on the carbon in the fifth position (C_5) of the sugar attaching to the upstream phosphate. The carbon in the sugar's third position (C_3) attaches to the downstream phosphate. Note that the 5′ terminus of this tetra-nucleotide carries a negatively charged phosphate group (P(–)), whereas the 3′ terminus ends on the sugar's hydroxyl group (OH). C_1 attaches to the base, and whether C_2 carries or does not carry a hydroxyl group distinguishes ribose (RNA) from deoxyribose (DNA), respectively.

quences, generating proteins or enzymes. The process of converting mRNA into protein is called **translation**.

A sequence of three nucleotides, usually abbreviated as its three-base sequence, is called a **codon** and corresponds to a specific amino acid (e.g.,

CGA corresponds to arginine), with the exception of **stop codons**, which provide a signal to terminate translation at the end of a gene sequence. (The 3-base-pair sequence complementary to a codon is an **anticodon**; for example, CAU is the anticodon for AUG.) In this way, an RNA sequence encodes a series of amino acids that, when linked together in series, create a distinct protein. Therefore, through this **central dogma of molecular biology**, the genetic information in genes is converted, or expressed, into proteins through a two-step process: from DNA to mRNA via transcription, then from mRNA to protein via translation. Expressed proteins then help determine the traits of the individual.

The largest units of DNA are chromosomes. Humans carry 23 pairs of chromosomes (22 **autosomes** and one **sex chromosome**), typically obtaining one copy of each chromosome from each parent. One gene can vary in its sequence because of an inherited difference or **de novo** (new) **mutation**. Each gene can have different variants or genetic differences, called **alleles**. The particular allele or combination of alleles that an individual carries is referred to as their **genotype**. Variation in the genetic sequence of an allele may lead to differences in the rate of gene **expression**, differences in the structure of the translated protein, or no functional difference at all, depending on how the nucleotide sequence has been changed. Each individual usually has two copies, or alleles, of each gene, and the phenotype is driven by the interaction of these two copies.

It is important to note that not all bases within the coding gene are translated into protein. A gene can contain a number of **exons** (coding sequences) and **introns** (noncoding). A process of posttranscriptional modification, or **splicing**, of the mRNA removes the introns, leaving only the merged exons to be translated into proteins (see Figure 1–2).

A process of condensation and organization is necessary to contain the enormous genome within the confines of the cell nucleus, as well as provide a mechanism for regulating gene expression. DNA is packaged, or condensed, into various levels of organization by interaction with proteins, yielding a structure called **chromatin** (see Figure 1–3). Proteins particularly important to this process are **histones**. DNA winds around octamers of core histones (specifically an assortment of H2A, H2B, H3, and H4) to form complexes known as **nucleosomes**. The interaction between histones and DNA is enhanced by charge differences. DNA is negatively charged owing to its phosphate backbone, and histone proteins are mostly positively charged owing to their high content of positively charged amino acids, including histidine, lysine, and arginine. Hydrophobic interactions provided by the methylated segments of the histone proteins also help in stabilizing the nucleosome complex. Like that of other

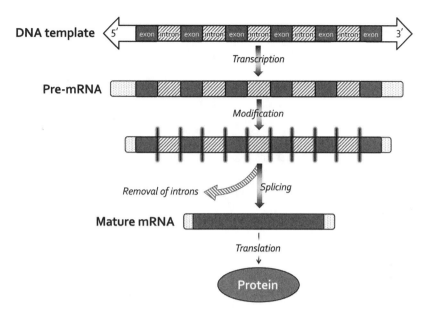

Figure 1–2. Posttranscriptional modification: overview of RNA splicing.

DNA forms a template that undergoes transcription to become RNA. This RNA is a precursor to mRNA (**pre-mRNA**) and must undergo modification before becoming mature, translatable mRNA. The modification process includes splicing, by which introns are removed and some or all of the exons remain. This final mature mRNA may then be translated into a protein.

nucleoproteins, histone interaction with DNA is sensitive to factors such as ionic strength, pH, presence of metal ions, and temperature (Andrews and Luger 2011). Additional nonhistone proteins also play a role in maintaining the chromatin structure, while others help regulate gene expression.

These opposing forces stabilize the nucleosome complex. Each nucleosome is bound by a linker histone (H1 or H5) and connected to the next nucleosome by linker DNA. These interactions give rise to the most lightly packed chromatin structure, named **euchromatin**, often compared to beads on a string. Linker histones allow further coiling to create chromatin fibers, creating a more condensed—and less transcriptionally active—chromatin structure called **heterochromatin**. This process of **chromatin remodeling** is dynamic, reversible, and crucial for regulation of gene expression. As is discussed later (see Histone Modification, page 21), each histone can be modified by methylation, acetylation, phosphorylation, ADP-ribosylation, or glycosylation, leading to an alter-

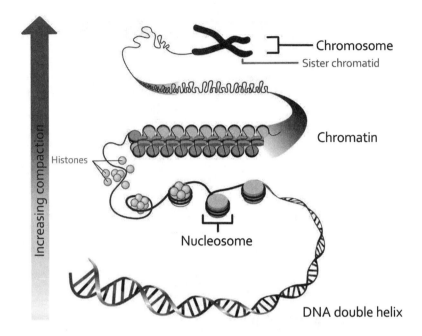

Figure 1–3.   DNA condensation.

DNA is packaged at a variety of levels, creating a reversibly condensed structure. At the first level, negatively charged DNA wraps around the mostly positively charged histone octamers to create stable nucleosomes. The series of linked nucleosomes are termed euchromatin and resemble beads on a string. Further coiling leads to a more condensed structure known as heterochromatin, the most condensed of which occurs only during cell replication and gametogenesis. In general, more stable nucleosomes and more condensed chromatin are associated with downregulation of the genes found in those regions.

Source.   Based on an image courtesy of the National Human Genome Research Institute (https://www.genome.gov/).

ation in net charge and shape of the nucleosome complex that may ultimately influence the regulation of expression of the genes tied to that particular nucleosome.

Conventional Nomenclature

As discussed above, the genome comprises a series of bases linked to a backbone of sugar and phosphate groups chained together. This chain has directionality that is recognized by transcriptional and translational machinery. Conventionally, we refer to this directionality as 5′ to 3′, indicating a forward direction, and 3′ to 5′, indicating a backward direction. The numbers refer to the numbering of carbon atoms in the base sugar, where the carbon in the 5' position links to the previous (**upstream**) phosphate group, and the carbon in the 3' position links to the next (**downstream**) phosphate group. Unless otherwise stated, descriptions of DNA base sequences are presented in a 5'-to-3' manner.

The nomenclature describing sections of the genome is based on the physical location of the specific locus with respect to chromosome, arm, and position (position is named relative to bands made visible through cytogenetic staining). The number or letter at the beginning of the name refers to the chromosome. After the number is either **p**, which refers to the short arm coming off the centromere, or **q**, which refers to the long arm. Next come numbers that indicate the region, band, and subband (see Figure 1–4). Therefore, **15q11-q13** (a section of particular importance for Prader-Willi and Angelman syndromes, among others, discussed further in Chapter 3, "Epigenetics in Neurodevelopmental and Neurodegenerative Disorders") refers to the area of chromosome 15's long arm, close to the centromere at region 1, covering bands 1–3.

Genes often have names that are similar, if not identical, to the protein they encode and typically are abbreviated with an alphanumeric moniker in italic type. Because human genes are often synonymous with analogous genes or proteins from rodent models, by convention, the abbreviation for the human gene is typically all uppercase (e.g., brain-derived neurotrophic factor [*BDNF*]), but only the first letter is uppercase in the abbreviation for the rodent gene (*Bdnf*). When referring to the protein, whether human or rodent, the abbreviation is written in all capitals roman type (BDNF). These conventions are followed throughout this book.

Epigenetics and Epigenetic Modifications

Epigenetics in a concise definition is the study of how the genome may be differently expressed without any alteration to the DNA base sequence. Through the lifelong course of development, epigenetic mechanisms are at play and are particularly crucial for cell cycle control, cell differentiation, cell growth, and the pathogenesis of certain diseases, including psychiatric disorders. A large portion of epigenetic modifications involve the addition of a molecule to DNA or histones, thus affecting a gene's ability to interact with transcriptional machinery. Specifically, a neutral, hydrophobic organic molecule (a methyl group, CH_3) may be added to select portions of DNA or histones (methylation), or a negatively charged molecule (an acetyl group, $-CO-CH_3$, or a phosphate group, $-PO_4$) may be added to histones (acetylation and phosphorylation, respectively). These

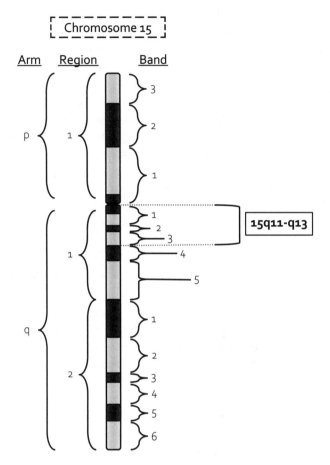

Figure 1–4.   Genome region naming.

Chromosome naming based on arm, region, and band. In this example, chromo-some 15 has one region in the p arm and two regions in the q arm. Within these regions, there are varying bands. Not pictured here are subbands, which are smaller classifications within bands denoted by a number after a decimal point. The convention for naming a particular section is to start with the number or letter of the chromosome followed by the arm, region, and band. 15q11-q13 denotes a section including bands 1–3 of region 1 on arm q of chromosome 15.

additions can affect how DNA interacts with **promoters** or how tightly DNA is compacted, thus affecting the expression of the gene without al-tering the DNA sequence. The sum total of these epigenetic markings in an individual is referred to as the **epigenome**. Additional mechanisms important to epigenetics in the body include the function of **noncoding RNA** and **microRNAs** (small regulatory RNAs often denoted **miRNAs**).

	Positive environment	Moderate stress	Chronic stress environment
Protective allele	Typical phenotype	Typical phenotype	Diseased phenotype
Risk allele	Typical phenotype	Diseased phenotype	Diseased phenotype

Figure 1–5. Interaction of environment and genetic predisposition.

Hypothetical representation of possible outcomes resulting from the varied combination of allele types and environmental stressors. Significant, chronic stress may yield a diseased phenotype regardless of genetic predisposition, whereas moderate stress may evoke pathology in individuals carrying risk alleles, but not in those with protective alleles.

Importantly, epigenetic changes may occur in response to an environmental trigger, may persist for a short or long time, and in some cases may be transmitted to offspring. In this way, the rate of gene expression can be affected by environmental factors.

Epigenetic modifications may be triggered by environmental stimuli and experiences, but it is also important to note that individuals carry varying degrees of genetic vulnerability that affect how likely epigenetic change is, or in turn how likely pathology is to emerge if epigenetic change does occur (see Figure 1–5). This relationship becomes crucial in applications of genetics and epigenetics to psychiatry, such as in cases of trauma and chronic stress (see Figure 1–6), which is the focus of Chapter 4, "Epigenetics of Childhood Trauma and Resilience," and in the development of psychopharmacological interventions.

Gene Promoters

To consider the mechanisms of epigenetics, it is important to review pertinent details of how gene transcription occurs. **RNA polymerase II (Pol**

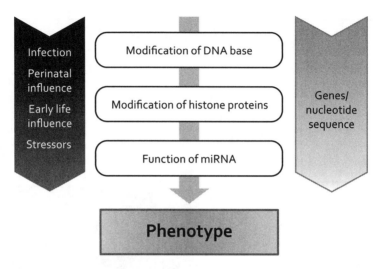

Figure 1–6. Overview of epigenetic interplay between genes and environment.

Epigenetic modifications are driven by the interplay between genes and the environment, and these changes impact phenotypes. Environmental events—such as perinatal and early life influence, infection, and stressors—dynamically interact with underlying genetic vulnerabilities via epigenetic mechanisms including modifications of DNA bases (including attachment of methyl groups), modifications of histones, and function of miRNAs. Some allele forms may be more vulnerable than others to certain epigenetic modifications.

II) is the complex that transcribes a gene to RNA. The resulting RNA transcript may yield a non-protein-coding transcript or a precursor to mRNA that then undergoes translation to become a protein. Pol II, however, cannot bind to DNA without the help of additional proteins called **transcription factors** (Haberle and Stark 2018). Gene promoters are nucleotide sequences along the genome where Pol II may assemble with transcription factors to create a **preinitiation complex**, allowing for initiation of the transcription process (see Figure 1–7). Once transcription starts, most of the preinitiation complex is left behind, while Pol II continues elongating the transcribed RNA based on the DNA sequence of the gene until a termination signal is reached. Structurally, the promoter is divided into three major segments: **core promoter**, **proximal promoter**, and **distal promoter**. The core segment is the site of assembly of the preinitiation complex. Various core promoters have been analyzed, with some being classified as focused, sharp, or single-peak promoters and others as broad or dispersed-peak promoters (Müller et al. 2007). The single-peak pro-

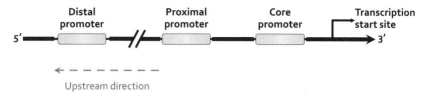

Figure 1–7. Overview of promoter structures.

Gene promoters are nucleotide sequences that lie upstream from the transcription start site, which is the beginning of the coding region. The promoter is divided into three major segments: the core promoter, the proximal promoter, and the distal promoter. The core promoter is relevant for staging the preinitiation complex; the proximal promoter contains regulatory sequences, particularly CpG islands; and the distal promoter (located much farther upstream) includes further regulatory sequences including enhancers, insulators, and silencers.

moters have a tightly defined transcription start site, may include TATA box or initiator motifs, and are more likely to contain transcription factor binding sites. In comparison, broad core promoters have a relatively less defined transcription start site and are less likely to contain transcription factor binding sites. In addition, the broad core promoters are often associated with **CpG islands** (see next section) and are more involved in the regulation of genes expressed ubiquitously across multiple tissue types.

Upstream of the core promoter segment is the proximal promoter segment. It includes several patterns of nucleotides such as CpG islands and sequences, which create binding sites for transcription factors, including the GC box and *cis*-regulatory modules. CpG islands are concentrated in the proximal promoter region. The distal part of the promoter region is upstream of the proximal promoter and contains entities such as enhancers, insulators, and silencers (Kumar and Bansal 2018).

CpG Islands

CpG islands are made of sequences of ~1,000 base pairs containing an elevated proportion of cytosine-[phosphate]-guanine (CG or CpG) dinucleotides, where the cytosine is frequently unmethylated. Generally speaking, vertebrates are devoid of CpG dinucleotide repeats, in part because cytosine in the CpG islands, once methylated, is susceptible to spontaneous deamination, causing the base to mutate into thymine, which could cause disruption of the normal function of the gene or its transcript. That said, the human genome is robustly punctuated with CpG islands, which are mostly unmethylated and thus avoid **mutation**. Although the majority of the CpG islands in vertebrates are unmethylated, a fundamental finding of epigenetics is that control of gene expression is affected by differential methylation at the CpG islands (Deaton and Bird 2011).

Around half of CpG islands are found within the promoter region, particularly the proximal promoter region. The remaining half of CpG islands, outside the gene promoter regions, are known as **orphan CpG islands**. Orphan CpG islands are classified as either **intragenic** (found within genes) or **intergenic** (found between genes). The orphan CpG islands exhibit promoter function and hence regulate transcriptional activity in the context of genomic **imprinting**, development, and cell differentiation (Deaton and Bird 2011; Sarda and Hannenhalli 2018).

Gene Regulation

Since the start of the Human Genome Project, data have been gathered to better quantify the number of genes contained within the human genome. After the first complete draft of the human genome, the estimate was 20,000–25,000 protein-coding genes; more recent estimates have narrowed the range to ~20,000 protein-coding genes and 22,000 noncoding genes (Pertea and Salzberg 2010; Pertea et al. 2018). This great volume of genes undergoing transcription and translation to maintain adequate gene expression requires extensive energy, highlighting the need for efficient gene regulation. Therefore, to not overexpend metabolic resources, there must be a conservative way of promoting the expression of needed genes while suppressing the expression of those that are not needed at that time.

Tight gene regulation is also needed for precise management of cellular processes. One example of the power of well-orchestrated gene regulation is the differentiation of stem cells. In a complex multicellular organism, all stem cells carry similar genomic sequences, but as they differentiate into various cell lines (skin, muscle, liver, etc.), certain genes are turned on, or expressed, while others are turned off, or silenced (see Figure 1–8). The different combinations of expressed and silenced genes determine which cell line is formed. Therefore, the process of gene regulation is crucial for stem cell differentiation, among other vital biological processes.

Levels of Gene Regulation

Transcriptional Level

In transcription, the first step described by the central dogma of molecular biology, the information contained in the DNA is copied (or tran-

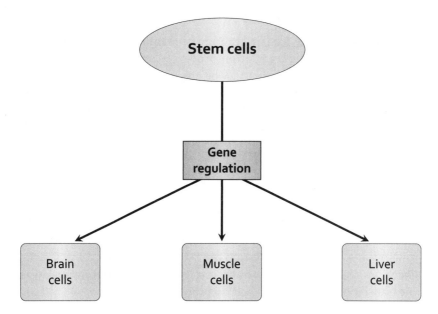

Figure 1–8. Gene regulation in stem cell differentiation.

All stem cells contain similar genomic sequences but differentiate into functionally different cell lines. This is possible with tight regulation of what combinations of genes are turned on and off.

scribed) into RNA. This process requires the DNA sequence itself and other factors such as transcription factors, replication enzymes, and non-protein-coding RNA. Gene expression can therefore be affected at this level by interference with the binding of transcription factors or replication enzymes, differences in the DNA sequence, or regulation of non-protein-coding RNAs.

Transcription factors themselves may contribute to gene regulation. General transcription factors bind within the core promoter region; other transcription factors bound at distant enhancers are able to interact with general transcription factors because the intervening DNA can form loops, bridging the gap and enhancing the interaction. These interactions at the promoter region help to regulate the function of the replication enzymes, thus affecting gene expression. CpG islands in the proximal promoter region also serve as a genomic platform in the process of gene regulation at the transcriptional level. Methylation of CpG islands and other local chromatin structural changes, such as chromatin remodeling, are proposed mechanisms of epigenetic transcriptional regulation (Deaton and Bird 2011).

Posttranscriptional Level

Processing of the RNA transcript to a mature mRNA can include splicing in preparation for the translation process. **Alternative splicing**—in which the same gene transcript may be processed in different ways, for example, by omitting one or more exons—is a regulatory instance that may yield different mRNA isoforms. The mRNA can also be targeted by miRNAs, leading to interference with the translation process or even destruction of the mRNA.

Translational Level

During translation, the second step described by the central dogma of molecular biology, ribosomes in the cytoplasm or endoplasmic reticulum alongside other substrates drive the process of protein synthesis from the mRNA transcript. Gene expression can be altered at this level by interference with some of these substrates, evoking subsequent termination of the translational process and halting protein synthesis.

Posttranslational Level

Regulation at the posttranslational level involves modification of the translated protein in such a way that its function is altered. One example is the cleavage of **pro-BDNF**, a precursor to mature BDNF protein that is necessary to produce a functional BDNF protein. Additional posttranslational modifications come in the form of enzymatic additions of chemical groups to proteins, such as the attachment of methyl or acetyl groups to histones, which may alter function.

DNA Methylation

In eukaryotes, DNA methylation occurs primarily on cytosine bases. The methylation step is carried out by a **DNA methyltransferase (DNMT)** enzyme in the presence of a methyl group donor (primarily *s*-**adenosyl-methionine**, known as SAM or SAM-e). During this process, the hydrogen on the carbon atom in the fifth position of the cytosine base is replaced with a methyl group, yielding 5-methylcytosine (5mC).

As described above, cytosine is densely concentrated into CpG islands or orphan CpG islands. Methylated orphan CpG islands regulate activity of genomic imprinting, development, and cell differentiation (Deaton and Bird 2011; Sarda and Hannenhalli 2018). The addition of methyl groups to DNA within the promoter region may induce gene silencing through a combination of proposed mechanisms (see Figures 1–9 and

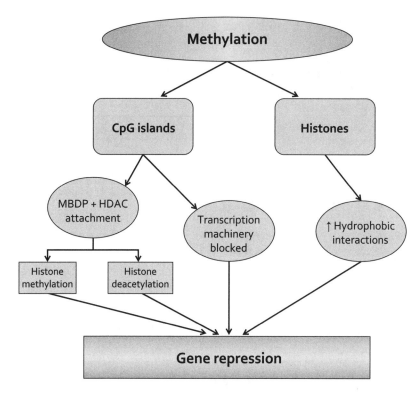

Figure 1–9. Mechanism of gene repression via methylation.

Methylation can occur in the CpG islands of the promoter region of a gene, inhibiting transcription. Methylation can also occur directly on histones, leading to increased hydrophobic interactions and further condensation of the chromatin structure.

↑=increased; CpG=cytosine-phosphate-guanine; HDAC=histone deacetylase; MBDP=**methyl-CpG-binding domain protein**.

1–10). First, the methyl group is nonpolar and thus provides a hydrophobic interaction within the genome, leading to more tightly packed chromatin. Second, methylation around the promoter region is postulated to directly prevent binding of the transcription machinery needed for gene transcription. Finally, methylated CpG segments can trigger the recruitment of other proteins, including **methyl CpG binding protein 2 (MeCP2)**, which is considered to exercise primarily downregulating activity, and chromatin remodeling complexes. Chromatin remodeling complexes that carry a methyl-CpG-binding domain can bind to methylated CpG sites and greatly alter the structure of the nucleosome, affecting associated gene expression (Hoffmann and Spengler 2019).

A. Unmethylated CpG islands

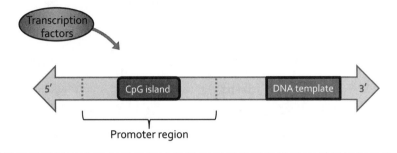

Promoter region

- -

B. Methylated CpG islands

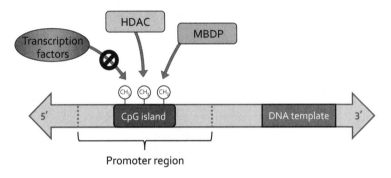

Promoter region

Figure 1–10. Methylation of CpG islands.

Gene repression occurs via methylation of CpG islands on the DNA template. (**A**) In unmethylated CpG islands, transcription factors and DNA replication enzymes may bind to the promoter region, thus allowing transcription to take place. (**B**) In methylated CpG islands, transcription factors and DNA replication enzymes are less able to interact with the promoter region, thereby downregulating transcription. In addition, recruitment of MBDP and HDAC leads to deacetylation and methylation of histone tails.

CH3=methyl group bound to cytosine bases; CpG=cytosine-phosphate-guanine; HDAC=histone deacetylase; MBDP=methyl-CpG-binding domain protein.

Determining DNA Methylation

DNA methylation patterns are examined in different ways, and it is important when approaching the literature to take note of the manner in which DNA methylation was quantified. One point of differentiation is whether a study indicates the specific sites of methylation or rather presents more general methylation patterns. Non-site-specific, global methylation across the entire genome may be determined directly by genomewide analysis, which calculates the ratio of methylated to total cytosine (Vryer and Saffery 2017). From this value, it may be determined whether the sample was globally hypermethylated, hypomethylated, or equivalent versus a comparison group. Another, more indirect, method restricts the search to sites considered to be representative of the entire genome, a common example being **long interspersed element 1 (LINE-1)**. It is important to note that these metrics of generalized hypermethylation or hypomethylation do not imply that the same pattern will hold for specific genes.

On the other hand, some studies presenting data on the spatial distribution of DNA methylation are better able to specifically define where the changes occur, allowing for further inferences about how the differences in presence or absence of DNA methylation may affect gene regulation mechanisms. A greater presence of DNA methylation at a particular site on the genome may be associated with reduced expression or silencing of a gene, but not always, so it is important to establish a correlation with downstream effects, such as indicators of protein expression.

Research examining the spatial distribution of methylated cytosine has become more common in applied studies of psychiatry. Many studies have focused on several genes previously implicated in genetic studies as having a role in the development of various mental health conditions. For example, research previously identified the serotonin transporter gene (*SLC6A4*) and *BDNF* as having potential roles in the development of major depressive disorder, and they have since been investigated with respect to their methylation patterns in the population with depression (see Chapter 2, "Epigenetic Modulation in Major Depressive Disorder"). In this way, the majority of studies of epigenetics in psychiatry have investigated specific genes chosen for their theorized relationship to certain disorders. Limiting studies to one gene or region of interest at a time has been mostly out of necessity, as characterizing the sheer immensity of data stored in the entire epigenome had previously not been feasible—or even possible—because of high costs, time demands, and the complexity of such massive data analyses. Over the past few decades, however, great advancements in laboratory techniques and data processing methodologies have allowed for more and more studies to examine methylation patterns of the entire genome at once.

The field of epigenetics has moved away from nonspecific global methylation patterns and single-gene approaches toward genomewide profiling of DNA methylation patterns, available down to single-base resolution. Techniques to analyze the entire genome—and epigenome—have come a long way since the renowned Human Genome Project began in 1990. One technique at the heart of that project was sequencing via chain termination, commonly referred to as Sanger sequencing. Sanger sequencing uses the target DNA sample as a template to make many partial copies at variable lengths, which are then used to determine the base sequence of the DNA sample. Sanger sequencing is still used at small scales, but large-scale applications have adopted techniques that are similar in concept but are capable of sequencing multiple DNA samples simultaneously. These methods are commonly referred to as **next-generation sequencing** (**NGS** or next-gen; also called second-generation sequencing or massive parallel sequencing). These advances in technology have been commercially available for >15 years, and research in the field of psychiatry has been gradually adopting them. A majority of the existing research in epigenetics applied to psychiatry has thus far used general global methylation patterns and single-gene approaches, and therefore this book mostly focuses on such studies. However, as the field continues to move forward, it is reasonable to anticipate that more research will use approaches to characterize genomewide methylation profiles.

This book is not intended to cover the nuanced details of research methods in epigenetics, but we present a brief overview of how genomewide methylation is typically performed. Although there are many different proprietary protocols and techniques, they share a general process of NGS. DNA is extracted from a sample and broken down into smaller fragments, through the use of either ultrasound (sonication), which breaks the DNA at random places, yielding fragments of length proportional to the time of exposure, or enzymes, which cleave DNA at more predictable sites. With the help of **primers**—short, single strands of nucleic acid that start DNA synthesis—the single-stranded DNA fragments are then washed over a plate of wells to which the DNA fragments may attach, with one DNA fragment per well. Once the assortment of single-stranded DNA fragments have been separated and immobilized, the apparatus is exposed to components and conditions required for DNA synthesis (including DNA polymerase as in Sanger sequencing). Instead of building one copy at a time as in Sanger sequencing, however, NGS builds millions of copies at once. The complementary strands for each of the DNA fragments are thus artificially synthesized while being closely monitored at each step. Data recorded during this phase reveal the DNA sequences of the complementary strands synthesized, which are then combined and processed through specialized computational programs.

Through NGS, DNA of a sample may now be sequenced relatively rapidly; the same technology can be adapted to also map methylation over the genome through **bisulfite sequencing**, in which methylated and unmethylated cytosine bases are differentiated through the process of bisulfite conversion. In the presence of sodium bisulfite, the unmethylated cytosine residues of a DNA sample convert to uracil, whereas the methylated cytosines (and the other bases) remain unchanged. During the sequencing step, these unmethylated Cs (now Us) are read as Ts. By comparing the output to known standards, the location of unmethylated Cs (presenting as Ts in the output) may be distinguished from methylated Cs (Cs in the output). In other words, if a thymine is found where a cytosine should be in the output, it is an unmethylated cytosine, and if a cytosine is found where it should be, it is a methylated cytosine.

Global methylation patterns determine only the proportion of cytosines that are methylated, providing a ratio of methylated to unmethylated cytosine across a given region, without specific information about where the methylated cytosines are located in the DNA sequence. Base-specific genomewide methylation profiles, on the other hand, reveal the precise locations of methylated cytosine across the entire genome. With advances in technology—in terms of both sequencing the DNA more rapidly and analyzing the massive datasets produced—the cost and time required for such analysis are now reasonable.

A final method for characterizing DNA methylation, which lies at the intersection of global methylation estimation and sequencing, is the use of **microarrays**. Research applications for microarrays are growing, as they provide a streamlined approach to characterizing methylation patterns in regions of interest across the genome. Instead of sequencing the entire genome or regions of interest, as with NGS, analysis via microarray uses differential methylation hybridization. A prepared, fragmented DNA sample is washed over a chip containing a library of DNA probes. If the sample contains complementary strands, those portions of the sample then bind or hybridize to the probes, and the binding strength of the sample to the known DNA probes is measured. As such, the data output from a DNA methylation microarray indicates the proportion of methylated cytosines for a given region of interest on the genome. DNA probes cover a significant portion of known sites of interest on the epigenome, including CpG islands, coding regions, promoters, and enhancers. The libraries of probes are proprietary; an example is the Infinium MethylationEPIC BeadChip, which includes probes spanning >850,000 CpG methylation sites (Moran et al. 2016). The spatial resolution of microarrays is therefore targeted and much more specific than global methylation analysis, but less specific than NGS (which can tell you down to the base sequence which cytosines are methylated across the entire genome).

Not only does the use of microarrays help to identify novel regions of interest, but it also allows DNA differences over multiple specific regions of the genome to be considered simultaneously. This may be done in different ways: some studies seek patterns directly in samples, and others compare DNA methylation patterns of samples to known networks, or gene sets, in a process called **enrichment analysis**. As data continue to be collected, large patterns—or networks—of regions of interest appear to commonly vary together: that is, differences in methylation in one area seem to frequently co-occur with differences in methylation of others, often in the region of known genes. Such patterns of gene sets are commonly tied to general biological processes, such as metabolism, neural synapse function, and neurodevelopment. These patterns over networks may then be examined in relation to a clinical sample to determine whether patterns of DNA methylation of the sample align with other patterns previously identified. As with NGS and microarrays, these types of analysis are massively complex and require intensive computational resources, all of which are subject to frequent development and expansion.

There are many nuances to these research methods, with different protocols, frequent updates, and adaptations moving them forward. Advancements in lab bench machines, microarray arrangements, and computational approaches also drive updates. Within medical applications of epigenetics, cancer research has consistently led in adopting new epigenetic research methods and study designs, therefore modeling useful techniques that may be adopted in other fields, including psychiatry.

Considerations for Approaching Current Literature

In approaching epigenetic research of DNA methylation, it is important to consider the sample source. Two major factors stand out: human versus animal models and direct tissue versus surrogate tissue sampling.

With respect to the organism sampled, animal models (frequently rodent models) allow for invasive studies that would be limited by sample size or ethical considerations if attempted in humans. In psychiatry, animals may perform behaviors or complete tasks in manners considered analogous to psychiatric diagnoses and neurobehavioral disorders. For example, a forced swim test may prompt a rodent to model learned helplessness in situations of despair; apathy may be demonstrated in features of nest building and self-grooming; and anxiety may be exhibited in avoiding open areas of the elevated plus maze (Becker et al. 2021). Although these models are elegant, overreliance on them can limit psychiatric applications, and so they are considered stepping stones to more focused clinical research with human populations.

In general, the most robust research examining DNA methylation focuses on samples taken from relevant tissue and demonstrates a relationship between the epigenetic marking pattern and consequent protein or RNA expression with clinical correlation. At this level of specificity, the tissue sampled can affect research findings. Often, DNA methylation patterns (and histone modifications, as discussed in the next section) are similar in blood cells and other specific tissues, allowing for an easily accessible sample source in humans. However, patterns of similarity between target tissues and their surrogates are gene and tissue specific, and thus peripheral blood samples do not always approximate the target tissue for a given parameter. Therefore, the use of peripheral blood as a surrogate source for a target tissue—neural tissue, for instance—must be done sparingly (see Bakulski et al. 2016 for a relevant review).

As a final note on DNA methylation, the majority of current research on epigenetic markings of DNA focuses on 5mC within CpG islands, but some exceptions are worth noting. First of all, methylation of cytosine also occurs at non-CpG sites, if methylated cytosine is followed in sequence by C, A, or T (Jang et al. 2017). Methylation of non-CpG sites appears to facilitate epigenetic regulation as well, with effects on neural development and correlates with neurodevelopmental disorders. Second, recent studies have demonstrated that 5mC may become oxidized by a ten-eleven translocation (TET) enzyme to form 5-hydroxymethylcytosine (5-hmC) (Richa and Sinha 2014). Research into this aspect of DNA hydroxymethylation has shown promising applications in cancer research (Zhu et al. 2020) as well as neurodevelopment and neurodegeneration (Szulwach et al. 2011; Zhao et al. 2017).

Histone Modification

Histone Methylation

Histone methylation involves the covalent linkage of a methyl group to arginine (R) or lysine (K) residues of the histone protein. Addition of a methyl group to a histone is facilitated by **histone methyltransferase (HMT)**; the removal of a methyl group is enabled by **histone demethylase**. Methylation can occur in various degrees such as monomethylation, dimethylation, or trimethylation. Each of these reversibly dynamic combinations can potentially alter chromatin structure, with subsequent effects on transcriptional activities. Histone modifications are named on the basis of the core histone, the specific residue affected, and how; for example, in histone 3 (H3), the lysine residue of the 27th position (K27) undergoing a trimethylation (me3) would be denoted H3K27me3.

Methylation of histone proteins does not necessarily alter the cationic charge, but it does increase hydrophobicity and steric bulk, especially when in the dimethylated or trimethylated state (Upadhyay and Cheng 2011). Methylation of neighboring histone proteins, depending on their proximity, may lead to hydrophobic folding of the genome. Although in general methylation is a hallmark for gene repression, methylation of specific lysine residues on histones has been shown to yield varying effects on transcription (Black et al. 2012). Specific examples include H3K27me3 and H3K9me3, which are generally associated with transcriptional repression, whereas H4K20me1, H3K36me3, H3K4me3, and H2BK5me1, among others, are associated with activation of transcription.

Histone Acetylation

Histone acetylation involves addition of the negatively charged acetyl group to a positively charged lysine residue of a histone protein. This covalent modification of histones exerts great influence on the transcriptional process. The mechanism through which histone acetylation affects gene expression may involve a charge effect, weakening the interaction between the DNA and histone protein, leading to a relaxation of the chromatin structure, and increasing the likelihood of transcription, as well as potentially signaling other factors to promote transcription (Verdone et al. 2006).

Histone acetylation is a reversible process catalyzed by **histone acetyltransferases (HATs)**, which yield addition of the acetyl group, and **histone deacetylases (HDACs)**, which allow removal of the acetyl group. These modifications are essential for cellular processes such as cell proliferation. As a result, it is not surprising that certain mutations or changes involving HATs could result in oncogenesis. The regulation of histone acetylation via exogenous HDAC inhibitors constitutes an area of research that may provide a novel therapeutic approach via regulation of gene expression. As such, the FDA has approved several HDAC inhibitors, including vorinostat and romidepsin, in the treatment of cancer (Kim and Bae 2011). The FDA has yet to approve HDAC inhibitors for other indications, but medications that have HDAC-inhibiting properties have been used in psychiatric contexts. In particular, the mood stabilizer and antiepileptic agent valproic acid has weak HDAC-inhibiting properties, which may contribute to its mechanism of action in psychiatric disorders (Machado-Vieira et al. 2011). Although this area of pharmacoepigenetics carries promising applications, the current state of treatment with HDAC inhibitors tends to be nonspecific and is associated with significant risks of side effects.

Histone Phosphorylation

The process of histone phosphorylation entails the addition of a phosphate group to serine, threonine, or tyrosine residues of the histone tail. This weakens the histone's interaction with DNA, destabilizing the nucleosome structure and typically increasing transcriptional activity. Phosphorylation is facilitated by protein kinases, whereas dephosphorylation is driven by phosphatases. In addition to affecting gene expression through chromatin compaction, histone phosphorylation plays a role in DNA damage repair, cell division, and a multitude of other cellular functions (Rossetto et al. 2012).

Imprinting

As a general rule, both parents contribute equally to the genetic makeup of their offspring, as each parent supplies one copy from each homologous chromosome pair to their child. This means that all offspring typically carry two copies of each chromosome, including each individual gene, which they inherit from both parents. In most cases, both gene copies (alleles) are expressed in the offspring. In some cases, however, **monoallelic expression** occurs, in which only one allele is expressed and the other is silenced (Ho-Shing and Dulac 2019).

An example of monoallelic expression comes from the process of genomic imprinting, the epigenetically controlled preferential expression of one parental allele over the other (Zink et al. 2018). This process involves methylation of a regulatory sequence of the gene or cluster of genes, thereby leading to molecular changes that may promote or prevent gene expression in some tissues based on the parent-of-origin. Several imprinted genes have been identified in humans, with mouse models suggesting >100–200 may exist. The known imprinted genes code for proteins as well as untranslated RNA transcripts (Bajrami and Spiroski 2016).

The process of **imprinting** begins during gametogenesis of both eggs and sperm, where genes may be tagged with epigenetic markers that follow a pattern indicating whether the parent-of-origin of the particular gene is the mother or father. After conception, the genes retain these epigenetic markers and may therefore be identified throughout the course of development and cell functioning based on which copy comes from the mother or father. Some genes in some tissues may then be imprinted if only one of the copies is expressed in a manner specific to the parent-of-origin. That is, if the maternal gene is imprinted, it is then silenced so that only the gene copy or allele from the father is expressed, which is thus known as a paternally expressed gene. If the paternal gene is imprinted, the allele from the mother is expressed and is referred to as a maternally expressed gene.

It is important to note that genes carrying the epigenetic patterns denoting parent-of-origin are not always expressed in a monoallelic fashion. Similarly, not all genes with monoallelic expression are due to imprinting. By definition, imprinting does not refer to the markers on the genes but rather the entire process of gene expression being regulated based on the parent-of-origin markers. This process may occur in a tissue-specific manner.

Whether an imprinted gene is expressed based on parent-of-origin relies heavily on the **imprinting control region (ICR)**, a sequence found on the chromosome near imprinted genes that regulates their expression. A common example of how the ICR works in a cluster of imprinted genes is the closely linked insulin-like growth factor 2 (*IGF2*) and *H19* genes (Ferguson-Smith and Bourc'his 2018; Yoshimizu et al. 2008). *H19* and *IGF2* neighbor closely enough to share enhancer elements, in addition to being reciprocally imprinted. Specifically, *IGF2* is typically maternally imprinted (silenced) so that the paternal allele is expressed, whereas *H19* is paternally imprinted and the maternal allele is expressed. A notable exception to this occurs in liver tissue, where *IGF2* imprinting becomes relaxed within the first year of postnatal life into adulthood, allowing alleles to be expressed from both parents simultaneously (**biallelic expression**) or monoallelically from either parent (Davies 1994; Ekström et al. 1995).

In tissues where *IGF2* and *H19* maintain their typical imprinting expression pattern, it has been proposed that the ICRs of these genes are generally methylated in the paternal allele and unmethylated in the maternal allele. The unmethylated ICR of the maternal allele binds to a particular transcription factor, CCCTC-binding factor (CTCF), which further enhances additional elements, ultimately leading to expression of the maternal *H19* allele (Pidsley et al. 2012). Simultaneously, the binding of CTCF mediates the assembly of chromatin insulators that interfere with *IGF2* promoter/enhancer interaction, thereby downregulating expression of the maternal *IGF2*. Because the paternal ICR is methylated, CTCF is unable to bind to this region, repressing *H19* expression. The absence of CTCF binding to the paternal allele then makes room for the interaction of promoter and enhancer elements of *IGF2*, facilitating the expression of *IGF2* in the paternal allele.

As discussed earlier, *IGF2* expression is favored when methylation is increased. This may seem counterintuitive, as methylation is generally considered a hallmark for gene repression. Although the methylation process mostly leads to a repressive state, in specific examples such as *IGF2*,

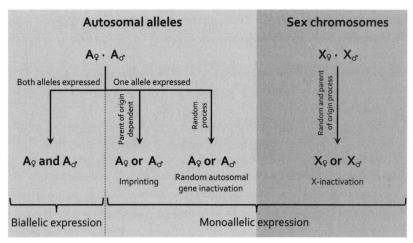

Figure 1–11. Allelic expression.

Except in the case of aneuploidy, every individual carries one copy of every chromosome from each parent. As a result, individuals typically carry two copies of each allele. Genetic and epigenetic mechanisms are in place to determine which genes will be expressed biallelically (both copies expressed simultaneously) or monoallelically (one allele silenced and the other expressed). The determination of which allele is silenced may occur randomly or epigenetically through imprinting. In the case of an individual with two X chromosomes, one is entirely inactivated through a combination of random and parent-of-origin–specific means, leading to monoallelic expression.

A♀=autosomal allele of maternal origin; A♂=autosomal allele of paternal origin; X♀=X chromosome of maternal origin; X♂=X chromosome of paternal origin.

methylation of both DNA and histone proteins could favor gene expression.

X-Inactivation

X-inactivation exemplifies epigenetic imprinting and monoallelic expression (see Figure 1–11). Except in cases of chromosomal duplication or loss, humans have 23 pairs of chromosomes, and one such pair is either two X chromosomes (usually female) or an X chromosome and a Y chromosome (usually male). This means there is a substantial difference in quantity—or dosage—of X-linked genes between individuals based on their chromosomes. X-inactivation is a process that serves to equilibrate this difference, which may be referred to as *dosage compensation*. In general, X-inactivation occurs in a rather complete way, such that one chromosome is selectively condensed into heterochromatin termed a *Barr body*. This marked condensation significantly decreases the likelihood of a gene on that chromosome being expressed. The process of X-inactivation is notably complex (see Borensztein et al. 2017; Disteche and Berletch 2015). Put simply, the process takes place through embryonic development and involves imprinting, but ultimately, whether the X chromosome of maternal or paternal origin is inactivated is largely random. However, the particular X chromosome that becomes inactivated is typically maintained over cell replication and therefore considered consistent across life.

The main concepts of X-inactivation may be exemplified in the fur pattern of domesticated cats, including calico and tortoiseshell cats. Tortoiseshell cats are (with rare exceptions as in the case of aneuploidy) always female and exhibit a coat of two colors, expressed in a mosaic pattern of dark brown and orange patches. This patchwork color display reflects underlying patterns of X-inactivation in the case where one X chromosome carries the allele for "orange" fur while the other carries the allele for "not orange" fur, producing the default, which in this case is blackish brown. From this common example, a few observations emerge that may be applied to the general understanding of X-inactivation. First, patches do not simultaneously express both the "orange" and "not orange" alleles, but rather they express one while the other is silenced. Second, patches do not change color under typical circumstances, suggesting that whichever X chromosome is active—whether of maternal or paternal origin—is relatively consistent in that cell line across the lifetime. Finally, the fur colors appear in patches rather than strands being entirely random and intermingled over the coat, suggesting that the pattern of X-inactivation may follow a mosaic pattern clustered spatially across tissues.

The mechanism by which X-inactivation occurs is rather complex, although it is understood to heavily involve **X-inactive specific transcript (*Xist*)** found within a region of the X chromosome known as the X-inactivation center (Brockdorff 2011; Wang et al. 2021). *Xist* is a DNA sequence that encodes a functional long noncoding RNA that plays a major role in recruiting and interacting with particular protein complexes and repressive epigenetic factors leading to chromatin compaction. During X-inactivation, upregulation of *Xist* occurs and is understood to, among other consequences, upregulate DNA methylation while increasing levels of the transcriptionally repressive methylated histones H3K9me2/H3K9me3 and H3K27me3 (Brinkman et al. 2006; Keniry et al. 2016) and also downregulating the transcriptionally activating acetylation of H3 and H4 plus trimethylation of H3K4 (Żylicz et al. 2019). Ultimately, these changes brought about by increased expression of *Xist* enhance the compaction of a select X chromosome into heterochromatin, effectively silencing genes of this condensed chromosome.

X-inactivation is an intricate, elegant mechanism that serves an important purpose; however, two related circumstances have emerged that may contribute to the development of pathology. First, despite the inactivated X chromosome undergoing considerable condensation, genes on it are sometimes able to be expressed, which is referred to as **X-inactivation escape**. The expression of these genes from the otherwise silenced X chromosome evokes a dose difference, which can lead to momentous phenotypic differences, with consequences ranging from various disease states to cell death. Examples include autoimmune diseases such as systemic lupus erythematosus, which is more prevalent in those with two X chromosomes and involves some genes that have escaped X-inactivation (Syrett et al. 2019). Second, a concept emerging in psychiatric epigenetic literature is **skewed X-inactivation**, in which the proportion of maternally versus paternally expressed X chromosomes is out of balance (Shvetsova et al. 2019). Skewed X-inactivation has been suggested to play a role in sex differences in symptomatology and incidence of disorders including schizophrenia (Zhang et al. 2020), intellectual disabilities (Plenge et al. 2002), and Alzheimer's disease (Bajic et al. 2015). Future research into the role of X-inactivation escape and skewed X-inactivation may further inform our understanding of sex differences in psychiatric disorders.

Noncoding RNAs

By definition, **noncoding RNAs** are strands of RNA that are not translated into a protein end-product. However, these strands of RNA serve a regulatory function at both the posttranscriptional and translational levels. There are various forms of regulatory noncoding RNAs, including the short noncoding RNAs—miRNAs, Piwi-interacting RNA, and small interfering RNA—and the long noncoding RNAs, such as *Xist* discussed previously. Substantial and growing evidence suggests that these regulatory RNAs play a substantial role in genomic epigenetic regulation (Wei et al. 2017).

miRNA

The final instrument of epigenetic regulation to be discussed here is microRNAs. Mature miRNAs are small and single stranded and comprise ~18–25 nucleotides. The molecules are either intergenic (transcribed independently from neighboring genes) or **intronic** (transcribed along with another gene before being excised during posttranscriptional modification) (Macfarlane and Murphy 2010). The primary miRNA transcript is initially processed to become the precursor miRNA (~70 nucleotides), which is then transported from the nucleus to the cytoplasm for further processing. In the cytoplasm, precursor miRNA is processed further by endonucleases to yield the final, mature miRNA. Functionally, mature miRNA can silence a gene either by degrading the mRNA transcript or by preventing the attachment of ribosomal subunits, thus interfering with the process of translation. This gene-silencing function of miRNAs has broad reach, affecting the regulation of developmental timing and the expression of genes in various disease states. Although miRNAs yield their own epigenetic effects on gene expression, they are also dynamically affected by other epigenetic mechanisms, such as DNA methylation and histone modification affecting their own expression (Gulyaeva and Kushlinskiy 2016; Yao et al. 2019).

Conclusion

Despite the complexities of epigenetics, a few principles repeatedly emerge across the clinical literature and within the field of psychiatry. In particular, patterns of DNA methylation, histone modification, and the role of noncoding RNA are frequently explored in relation to expression of mental health and psychiatric pathology. In the chapters to come, these mechanisms remain in the spotlight as we present relevant epigenetic research applied to mood disorders, neurodevelopmental and neurodegenerative disorders, trauma and resilience, and wellness and aging. It is our hope that the information presented here will provide a sufficient base of knowledge to allow readers to continue onward, comprehending new research and thoughtfully considering how emerging research may be applied to the clinical setting.

KEY POINTS

- Genetic information is stored within the deoxyribonucleic acid (DNA) inside the nucleus of the cell, and cannot leave. To be expressed, another temporary molecule, ribonucleic acid (RNA), is produced (through transcription) and used to carry the exact DNA sequence out of the nucleus into the body of the cell, where it either functions as a noncoding RNA or is translated into protein.

- Modification of gene products may occur after transcription (posttranscription) and/or after translation (posttranslation). An example of posttranscriptional modification is gene splicing, in which introns are removed, leaving only the merged exons to be translated into proteins. An example of posttranslational modification is cleavage of immature protein products to create mature, functional proteins.

- DNA winds around octamers of core histones to form complexes known as nucleosomes. Each nucleosome is bound by a linker histone and connected to the next nucleosome by linker DNA, resembling beads on a string, forming the most lightly packed (and typically more transcriptionally active) chromatin structure. Further coiling into more condensed structures may occur, creating more compaction into heterochromatin, which is considered less transcriptionally active. This process, known as chromatin remodeling, is dynamic, reversible, and crucial for regulation of gene expression.

- Epigenetics involves how gene expression can be changed without altering the DNA base sequence. Environmental mechanisms are susceptible to change in the context of environmental events. A large portion of epigenetic modifications involve the addition of a molecule to DNA or histones, affecting how DNA interacts with promoters, or how tightly DNA is compacted, thus affecting the expression of the gene without altering the DNA sequence. Additional relevant epigenetic mechanisms include the function of noncoding and microRNAs. Epigenetic changes may occur in response to an environmental trigger, may persist for a short or long time, and in some cases may be transmitted to offspring. In this way, the rate of gene expression can be affected by environmental factors.

- CpG islands in DNA are made of sequences of ~1,000 base pairs containing an elevated proportion of cytosine-[phosphate]-guanine (CG or CpG) dinucleotides, often in the promoter regions of genes. Control of gene expression is affected by differential methylation of DNA (via DNA methyltransferase [DNMT]), particularly at CpG islands. DNA methylation status may affect expression of the nearby gene by preventing binding of transcription machinery, more tightly packing chromatin, and triggering the recruitment of other proteins affecting gene expression and chromatin structure.

- Common histone modifications include methylation (often, but not always, downregulating expression), acetylation (upregulating expression), and phosphorylation (typically upregulating expression). Such modifications may be triggered by the environment and occur through particular enzyme reactions, which have been of interest as a potential target of therapeutic intervention (in particular, histone deacetylase [HDAC] inhibitors received approval by the FDA for the treatment of some cancers).

- Genomic imprinting is the epigenetically controlled preferential expression of one parental allele over the other. Imprinting does not refer to the marks on the genes but rather the entire process of gene expression being regulated based on the parent-of-origin markings.

- In individuals carrying two X chromosomes, X-inactivation occurs when one of the X chromosomes is markedly condensed in a manner that significantly decreases the likelihood of a gene on that chromosome being expressed. Whether the inactivated X chromosome is of maternal or paternal origin is largely random, although the selection is typically maintained consistently across the life span.

- RNA may perform functions, including epigenetic regulation, without being translated into proteins. These noncoding RNAs serve regulatory functions at the posttranscriptional and translational levels. MicroRNAs (miRNAs) are noncoding RNAs that can silence a gene either by degrading the mRNA transcript or by preventing attachment of ribosomal subunits, inhibiting translation.

Study Questions

1. The segment of DNA that may be encoded into a protein is termed

   A. Codon
   B. Anticodon
   C. Gene
   D. Promoter
   E. Nucleosome

   Best answer: C

   Explanation: A gene (answer C) is a DNA sequence that may be transcribed into noncoding RNA or coding RNA. A codon (answer A) is a three-base sequence that codes for a particular amino acid or signal to stop translation. For example, CAG is a codon that codes for the amino acid glutamine. An anticodon (answer B) is the complementary sequence of three base pairs to the codon; for example, CAU (5′ to 3′) is the anticodon for AUG. A protein comprises a series of amino acids; therefore, it requires a sequence of codons. A promoter region (answer D) is a nucleotide segment that lies upstream to a gene. The promoter serves multiple functions, as it provides the site for assembly of transcription enzymes and transcription factors, while also functioning in the regulation of gene expression. A nucleosome (answer E) is a DNA-histone complex and serves as the fundamental structural unit of the chromosome.

2. True or false: Cytosine-[phosphate]-guanine (CpG) islands that may undergo methylation are found exclusively within promoter regions.

   Best answer: False

   Explanation: Approximately half of CpG islands are found in promoter regions; the other half are considered orphan CpG islands, as they lie outside promoter regions. Orphan CpG islands are further classified into intragenic (within genes) and intergenic (between genes). Regardless of location, CpG islands are understood to be prone to methylation changes.

3. Which of the following is correct about imprinted genes?

   A. Both inherited alleles are always expressed
   B. Only one of the inherited alleles is usually expressed
   C. Imprinted genes are not inherited
   D. Usually, neither allele is expressed

   Best answer: B

   Explanation: For imprinted genes, usually only one allele (i.e., either the maternally or paternally inherited allele) is expressed (answer B). Recall that during gametogenesis, imprinted genes in both egg and sperm are identified and may be tagged with epigenetic marks allowing for differentiation after fertilization. If the maternal gene is imprinted, only the gene copy or allele from the father will be expressed. On the other hand, if the paternal gene is imprinted, only the allelic copy from the mother is expressed. Imprinted genes are inherited or transmitted from parents to offspring (contradicting answer C). As imprinting is an epigenetic silencing of one allele in a parent-of-origin manner, both alleles of an imprinted gene are not expected to be expressed (as in answer A). Cases in which neither allele is expressed (answer D) typically result in pathology or cell death.

4.   Which of the following describes monoallelic expression?

    A. An instance where only the maternal allele is expressed
    B. An instance where only the paternal allele is expressed
    C. An instance where both the maternal and paternal alleles are expressed at the same time
    D. An instance where neither the paternal nor maternal allele is expressed
    E. Options A and B are correct

Best answer: E

Explanation: Monoallelic expression occurs when only one allele is expressed, whether from the mother (answer A) or from the father (answer B). Common examples include X-inactivation and imprinting. Biallelic expression occurs when both maternal and paternal alleles are simultaneously expressed (answer C). Cases where neither allele is expressed (answer D) typically result in pathology or cell death.

5.   Where does methylation of CpG islands mostly occur within human DNA?

    A. The cytosine base
    B. The phosphate group
    C. The pyrimidine base
    D. The guanine base

Best answer: A

Explanation: DNA methylation typically takes place at the 5′ position of the cytosine base (answer A). In research, this is primarily recorded within CpG islands, although it is possible for cytosine to be methylated when followed by any other base. Guanine (answer D) and pyrimidines (answer C) other than cytosine (thymine in DNA and uracil in RNA) do not typically undergo methylation. The phosphate group (answer B) and pentose sugar linking the bases do not undergo methylation either. Phosphorylation of the genome at various histones can occur, and this is one of the various epigenetic modifications that could alter gene expression.

6. What is the typical effect of DNA methylation at the 5′ position of the cytosine base?

    A. No effect on gene expression
    B. Increased gene expression
    C. Drastic change in the base sequence of the genome
    D. Decreased gene expression

Best answer: D

Explanation: In general, methylation at the 5′ position of the cytosine base is a hallmark for gene repression (answer D). Hypermethylation of CpG islands is likely to interfere with gene expression (unlike answer A) by preventing the interaction of replication machinery with the promoter region. Also, hypermethylation may provide increased hydrophobic interaction within the genome, leading to more tightly packed chromatin. Alternatively, demethylation of DNA is more likely to enhance gene expression (answer B). DNA methylation of cytosine does not alter the base sequence of the genome (contradicting answer C). The epigenetic process itself does not lead to base-sequence alteration or mutation of the genome; however, methylated cytosine is more susceptible to spontaneous deamination, causing a mutation into thymine.

7. What is the effect of histone methylation on gene expression?

    A. Increased gene expression
    B. Decreased gene expression
    C. Generally decreased gene expression, with instances of increased gene expression
    D. No impact on gene expression

Best answer: C

Explanation: In general, histone methylation leads to decreased gene expression (unlike answers A and D). However, methylation of specific lysine residues on histones has been shown to yield varying effects on transcription (contradicting answer B). In some instances, histone methylation serves as an active mark associated with increased expression, as in methylated H4K20, H3K36, H3K4, and H2BK5.

8. Which of the following typically leads to an increase in gene expression?

    A. Stabilization of the nucleosome
    B. Chromatin compaction
    C. Histone methylation
    D. Histone acetylation

    Best answer: D

    Explanation: Because of its phosphate backbone, DNA is negatively charged, whereas histone proteins are mostly positively charged based on their amino acid composition. These opposing charges provide stability to the nucleosome complex that may be enhanced or weakened with various modifications to the histone, which is an essential mechanism within the study of epigenetics. Changes that destabilize the nucleosome—such as adding negatively charged acetyl or phosphate groups—allow for transcription to more readily occur, increasing gene expression. A more stable nucleosome (answer A), achieved sometimes through adding methyl groups, which may increase hydrophobic interactions (answer C), is typically associated with a decrease in transcriptional activity for those genes. Condensation and compaction of chromatin (answer B) typically leads to a decrease in accessibility of genes for transcription machinery, downregulating gene expression.

9. Which of the following regulatory mechanisms best depicts an epigenetic process?

    A. X chromosome inactivation
    B. Gene mutations
    C. RNA splicing
    D. Trinucleotide repeat expansion

    Best answer: A

    Explanation: X chromosome inactivation (answer D) is a process that serves to equilibrate the dosage differences in X-linked genes in those with two X chromosomes versus one X and one Y chromosome. The silencing of one X chromosome involves imprinting; whether the chromosome of maternal or paternal origin is inactivated is largely random. The silencing of one X chromosome occurs through significant condensation into heterochromatin. This process relies on the work of epigenetic machinery, including upregulation of DNA methylation and transcriptionally repressive histone methylation, with downregulation of transcriptionally activating histone acetylation. These processes do nothing to the DNA sequence of the X chromosome, which has been silenced. On the other hand, gene mutations (answer B) and trinucleotide repeat expansion (answer D) are consequences of genetic processes that lead to nucleotide sequence alteration. Trinucleotide repeat expansions (answer D), discussed in Chapter 3, "Epigenetics in Neurodevelopmental and Neurodegenerative Disorders, are related to genetic diseases including fragile X syndrome and Huntington's disease. RNA splicing (answer C) is an example of a posttranscriptional modification in which introns are removed from mRNA and exons remain in sequence before translation into a protein.

References

Andrews AJ, Luger K: Nucleosome structure(s) and stability: variations on a theme. Annu Rev Biophys 40(1):99–117, 2011 21332355

Bajic V, Mandusic V, Stefanova E, et al: Skewed X-chromosome inactivation in women affected by Alzheimer's disease. J Alzheimers Dis 43(4):1251–1259, 2015 25159673

Bajrami E, Spiroski M: Genomic imprinting. Open Access Maced J Med Sci 4(1):181–184, 2016 27275355

Bakulski KM, Halladay A, Hu VW, et al: Epigenetic research in neuropsychiatric disorders: the "tissue issue." Curr Behav Neurosci Rep 3(3):264–274, 2016 28093577

Becker M, Pinhasov A, Ornoy A: Animal models of depression: what can they teach us about the human disease? Diagnostics (Basel) 11(1):123, 2021 33466814

Black JC, Van Rechem C, Whetstine JR: Histone lysine methylation dynamics: establishment, regulation, and biological impact. Mol Cell 48(4):491–507, 2012 23200123

Borensztein M, Syx L, Ancelin K, et al: Xist-dependent imprinted X inactivation and the early developmental consequences of its failure. Nat Struct Mol Biol 24(3):226–233, 2017 28134930

Brinkman AB, Roelofsen T, Pennings SWC, et al: Histone modification patterns associated with the human X chromosome. EMBO Rep 7(6):628–634, 2006 16648823

Brockdorff N: Chromosome silencing mechanisms in X-chromosome inactivation: unknown unknowns. Development 138(23):5057–5065, 2011 22069184

Davies SM: Developmental regulation of genomic imprinting of the IGF2 gene in human liver. Cancer Res 54(10):2560–2562, 1994

Deaton AM, Bird A: CpG islands and the regulation of transcription. Genes Dev 25(10):1010–1022, 2011 21576262

Disteche CM, Berletch JB: X-chromosome inactivation and escape. J Genet 94(4):591–599, 2015 26690513

Ekström TJ, Cui H, Li X, Ohlsson R: Promoter-specific IGF2 imprinting status and its plasticity during human liver development. Development 121(2):309–316, 1995 7768174

Ferguson-Smith AC, Bourc'his D: The discovery and importance of genomic imprinting. eLife 7:e42368, 2018 30343680

Gulyaeva LF, Kushlinskiy NE: Regulatory mechanisms of microRNA expression. J Transl Med 14(1):143, 2016 27197967

Haberle V, Stark A: Eukaryotic core promoters and the functional basis of transcription initiation. Nat Rev Mol Cell Biol 19(10):621–637, 2018 29946135

Hoffmann A, Spengler D: Chromatin remodeling complex NuRD in neurodevelopment and neurodevelopmental disorders. Front Genet 10(Jul):682, 2019 31396263

Ho-Shing O, Dulac C: Influences of genomic imprinting on brain function and behavior. Curr Opin Behav Sci 25:66–76, 2019

Jang HS, Shin WJ, Lee JE, Do JT: CpG and non-CpG methylation in epigenetic gene regulation and brain function. Genes (Basel) 8(6):2–20, 2017 28545252

Keniry A, Gearing LJ, Jansz N, et al: Setdb1-mediated H3K9 methylation is enriched on the inactive X and plays a role in its epigenetic silencing. Epigenetics Chromatin 9(1):16, 2016 27195021

Kim HJ, Bae SC: Histone deacetylase inhibitors: molecular mechanisms of action and clinical trials as anti-cancer drugs. Am J Transl Res 3(2):166–179, 2011 21416059

Kumar A, Bansal M: Modulation of gene expression by gene architecture and promoter structure, in Bioinformatics in the Era of Post Genomics and Big Data. London, InTech, 2018, pp 37–54

Macfarlane L-A, Murphy PR: MicroRNA: biogenesis, function and role in cancer. Curr Genomics 11(7):537–561, 2010 21532838

Machado-Vieira R, Ibrahim L, Zarate CA Jr: Histone deacetylases and mood disorders: epigenetic programming in gene-environment interactions. CNS Neurosci Ther 17(6):699–704, 2011 20961400

Moran S, Arribas C, Esteller M: Validation of a DNA methylation microarray for 850,000 CpG sites of the human genome enriched in enhancer sequences. Epigenomics 8(3):389–399, 2016

Müller F, Demény MA, Tora L: New problems in RNA polymerase II transcription initiation: matching the diversity of core promoters with a variety of promoter recognition factors. J Biol Chem 282(20):14685–14689, 2007 17395580

Pertea M, Salzberg SL: Between a chicken and a grape: estimating the number of human genes. Genome Biol 11(5):206, 2010 20441615

Pertea M, Shumate A, Pertea G, et al: CHESS: a new human gene catalog curated from thousands of large-scale RNA sequencing experiments reveals extensive transcriptional noise. Genome Biol 19(1):208, 2018 30486838

Pidsley R, Fernandes C, Viana J, et al: DNA methylation at the Igf2/H19 imprinting control region is associated with cerebellum mass in outbred mice. Mol Brain 5(1):42, 2012 23216893

Plenge RM, Stevenson RA, Lubs HA, et al: Skewed X-chromosome inactivation is a common feature of X-linked mental retardation disorders. Am J Hum Genet 71(1):168–173, 2002 12068376

Richa R, Sinha RP: Hydroxymethylation of DNA: an epigenetic marker. EXCLI J 13:592–610, 2014 26417286

Rossetto D, Avvakumov N, Côté J: Histone phosphorylation: a chromatin modification involved in diverse nuclear events. Epigenetics 7(10):1098–1108, 2012 22948226

Sarda S, Hannenhalli S: Orphan CpG islands as alternative promoters. Transcription 9(3):171–176, 2018 29099304

Shvetsova E, Sofronova A, Monajemi R, et al: Skewed X-inactivation is common in the general female population. Eur J Hum Genet 27(3):455–465, 2019 30552425

Syrett CM, Paneru B, Sandoval-Heglund D, et al: Altered X-chromosome inactivation in T cells may promote sex-biased autoimmune diseases. JCI Insight 4(7):e126751, 2019 30944248

Szulwach KE, Li X, Li Y, et al: 5-hmC-mediated epigenetic dynamics during postnatal neurodevelopment and aging. Nat Neurosci 14(12):1607–1616, 2011 22037496

Upadhyay AK, Cheng X: Dynamics of histone lysine methylation: structures of methyl writers and erasers. Prog Drug Res 67:107–124, 2011 21141727

Verdone L, Agricola E, Caserta M, Di Mauro E: Histone acetylation in gene regulation. Brief Funct Genomics Proteomics 5(3):209–221, 2006 16877467

Vryer R, Saffery R: What's in a name? Context-dependent significance of 'global' methylation measures in human health and disease. Clin Epigenetics 9(1):2, 2017 28149330

Wang W, Min L, Qiu X, et al: Biological function of long non-coding RNA (lncRNA) Xist. Front Cell Dev Biol 9:645647, 2021 34178980

Wei JW, Huang K, Yang C, Kang CS: Non-coding RNAs as regulators in epigenetics (Review). Oncol Rep 37(1):3–9, 2017 27841002

Yao Q, Chen Y, Zhou X: The roles of microRNAs in epigenetic regulation. Curr Opin Chem Biol 51:11–17, 2019 30825741

Yoshimizu T, Miroglio A, Ripoche MA, et al: The H19 locus acts in vivo as a tumor suppressor. Proc Natl Acad Sci USA 105(34):12417–12422, 2008

Zhang X, Li Y, Ma L, et al: A new sex-specific underlying mechanism for female schizophrenia: accelerated skewed X chromosome inactivation. Biol Sex Differ 11(1):39, 2020 32680558

Zhao J, Zhu Y, Yang J, et al: A genome-wide profiling of brain DNA hydroxymethylation in Alzheimer's disease. Alzheimers Dement 13(6):674–688, 2017 28089213

Zhu H, Zhu H, Tian M, et al: DNA methylation and hydroxymethylation in cervical cancer: diagnosis, prognosis and treatment. Front Genet 11:347, 2020 32328088

Zink F, Magnusdottir DN, Magnusson OT, et al: Insights into imprinting from parent-of-origin phased methylomes and transcriptomes. Nat Genet 50(11):1542–1552, 2018 30349119

Żylicz JJ, Bousard A, Žumer K, et al: The implication of early chromatin changes in X chromosome inactivation. Cell 176(1–2):182–197.e23, 2019 30595450

Epigenetic Modulation in Major Depressive Disorder

Onoriode Edeh, M.D.
Kyle J. Rutledge, D.O., Ph.D.

Building on the content of Chapter 1, "Overview of Genetic and Epigenetic Mechanisms," the rest of this book shares applications for the principles of epigenetics within psychiatry. The aim is to reinforce those concepts while presenting the most robust findings to date within the field of epigenetics in psychiatry. Our first exploration, and the focus of this chapter, is major depressive disorder (MDD), for which a majority of the epigenetic work has looked into the role that **brain-derived neurotrophic factor (BDNF)** may play in the etiology of depression.

Excessive environmental stressors, including early developmental **trauma** and chronic **stress**, have been reliably shown to decrease cognitive function and induce depressive traits. These effects come from an array of biological mechanisms, namely an increase in the rate of apoptosis in conjunction with a reduction in BDNF expression and subsequent decreased neurogenesis. As such, aberrant BDNF expression has been associated with a variety of mental illnesses, including MDD. Duman et al. (1997) initially theorized that the association between environmental stressors and depression—as well as the largely elusive mechanism of antidepressant treatments—could be through intracellular modulation of neurotrophic factors such as BDNF. Data gathered since then support this theory and suggest that epigenetic changes of *BDNF* may steer this relationship. Dysregulated BDNF has also been tied to other brain pathology, such as amyotrophic lateral sclerosis (ALS), Parkinson's disease, Alzheimer's disease, and Huntington's disease, and to lack of neuroprotection following a cerebrovascular accident (see Nagahara and Tuszynski [2011] for a review).

BDNF Function and Characterization

BDNF, a neuronal growth factor, has been studied extensively in humans and animal models. The neurotrophin stimulates cell differentiation, development, plasticity, and synaptogenesis, as well as long-term potentiation (Hing et al. 2018). *BDNF* is widely expressed in the central nervous system and is found in excitatory neurons and glial cells, but not in inhibitory neurons.

BDNF has been found to interact with various receptors but is most well known to bind to **tropomyosin receptor kinase B (TrkB)** (alternatively known as tyrosine receptor kinase B or neurotrophic receptor tyrosine kinase 2 [NTRK2]). Upon binding extracellularly, BDNF-TrkB leads to a cascade of intracellular effects, involving cleavage of phosphatidylinositol bisphosphate into diacylglycerol (DAG) and inositol trisphosphate (IP3). IP3 stimulates receptors on smooth endoplasmic reticulum, promoting Ca^{2+} release into the cytoplasm. DAG together with Ca^{2+} activates protein kinase C, which then phosphorylates downstream substrates including DNA binding proteins and other proteins impacting gene expression that ultimately influence synaptic plasticity (see Figure 2–1). The BDNF-TrkB complex is also understood to initiate cellular responses through phosphoinositide 3-kinase and mitogen-activated protein kinase (to activate and enhance dendritic growth and branching) as well as through GTPases (to stimulate growth of neural fibers, that is, actin and myotubules).

The human gene *BDNF* has 11 exons with 9 functional tissue-specific promoters, thus leading to numerous different transcripts that are identical in function but tissue specific. The multiple combinations of exons, under the regulation of many different promoters, allow for numerous transcripts that can be regulated based on cell type, tissue region, and even environmental stimulus (Cattaneo et al. 2016). Transcripts derived from exons 2, 3, 4, 5, and 7 are mostly brain specific (Pruunsild et al. 2007). Although these numerous transcripts from the same gene vary in their mRNA sequence, their respective initial protein products (pre-pro-

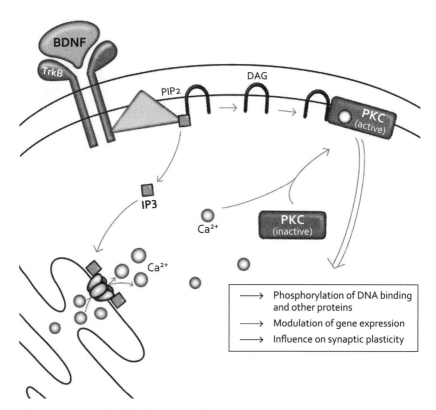

Figure 2–1.   BDNF-TrkB signaling pathways.

BDNF interacts with TrkB receptor, leading to a cascade of effects in the cell, with downstream effects on gene expression and synaptic plasticity. Not pictured here are further cellular effects of BDNF-TrkB through PI3K, MAPK, and GTPases.

Note.   BDNF=brain-derived neurotrophic factor; Ca^{2+}=calcium ion; DAG=diacylglycerol; IP3=inositol trisphosphate; MAPK=mitogen-activated protein kinase; PI3K=phosphoinositide 3 kinase; PIP2=phosphatidylinositol bisphosphate; PKC=protein kinase C; TrkB=tropomyosin receptor kinase B.

Source.   Image by Haley Rutledge, M.S.

BDNF) are cleaved to become the same BDNF precursor protein (pro-BDNF), which is further processed before ultimately yielding a mature BDNF protein that is identical across tissues.

An exception, however, is that BDNF structure and expression can vary across the population based on one or more alleles in an individual, as a result of **single-nucleotide polymorphisms (SNPs)**. Several *BDNF* SNPs have been found, with many studies demonstrating significant associations with the development of depression (Hing et al. 2018). One particularly well-studied polymorphism, Val66Met, results in a protein variant that differs by one amino acid—valine (Val) or methionine (Met)—at position 66 of pro-BDNF. In humans and animal models, those heterozygous or homozygous for the Met allele show decreased transcription and release of BDNF from neurons, which is associated with an increased vulnerability to early life adversity and increased risk for developing depression and anxiety (Ignácio et al. 2014).

BDNF Regulation in Major Depressive Disorder

Animal Models

MDD has a lower heritability than other psychiatric diagnoses, highlighting the significance of nongenetic factors in its development (Uchida et al. 2018). One such factor is environmental elements that modulate BDNF levels. The possible causal role of decreased BDNF protein levels leading to depression and cognitive decline has been supported by studies in which treatment with exogenous BDNF yields improvements in these same outcomes in rodents. Means of increasing endogenous levels of BDNF (e.g., through exercise, antidepressants, or ketamine) are also tied to reversal of stress-induced depression-like behaviors in rodents, decreased apoptosis, and increased neurogenesis (Hing et al. 2018).

Several epigenetic changes indicate potential mechanisms by which **toxic stress** can decrease BDNF expression in neural tissue (see Chapter 4, "Epigenetics of Childhood Trauma and Resilience," for more in-depth discussion of the effects of early toxic stress and trauma). In animal models, exposure to abusive parental care can lead to notable increases in DNA methylation at distinct *Bdnf* promoter regions, with associated decreased expression in the prefrontal cortex, and transmission to offspring (Roth et al. 2009). DNA methylation changes may occur as a result of stressors in utero as well, and these modifications could be further enhanced in the presence of parental care deficits (see Hing et al. [2018] for a review).

Beyond DNA methylation, histone modification may also influence BDNF expression through regulation of the wide variety of *Bdnf* mRNA transcripts. Modifications of the histones positioned at different exons of mouse *Bdnf* have been shown to vary across embryonic and postnatal development (Chen and Chen 2017). With the gene's numerous exons and promoters, differences in which *Bdnf* transcripts are expressed across different brain regions over developmental time points and extracellular or environmental stimuli—including pharmacological treatments—can change the specific transcripts predominantly found in these regions.

Histone modifications, which can regulate transcription at different exons by interactions with promoters and enhancers, may in part drive these differences in BDNF expression of neural tissue across developmental time points.

Clinical Populations

In addition to animal models, DNA hypermethylation has been associated with depressive phenotypes in human clinical studies (see Lockwood et al. [2015] for a systematic review). Adults with MDD have been noted to demonstrate increased DNA methylation in the *BDNF* promoter compared with unaffected control subjects (excluding individuals taking medications such as lithium and antipsychotics) (Roy et al. 2017). DNA methylation of the *BDNF* promoter has also been found to be significantly higher in patients with MDD and bipolar II disorder than in patients with bipolar I disorder or unaffected control subjects, suggesting different epigenetic patterns among separate affective disorders (Dell'Osso et al. 2014).

One longitudinal study examining depression in women with breast cancer following mastectomy underscored this relationship between *BDNF* methylation and depression (Kang et al. 2015). Women were evaluated 1 week after mastectomy and again 1 year later for diagnosis of MDD and severity classification. The methylation status of one cytosine-[phosphate]-guanine dinucleotide (CpG) island within the *BDNF* promoter taken from peripheral blood samples was then compared across MDD status and severity. Results showed a strong association between *BDNF* promoter methylation status and depression diagnosis both 1 week and 1 year after breast cancer surgery.

Neuroanatomical correlates of *BDNF* methylation and depression have also been demonstrated. One of the first studies to highlight this relationship used DNA extracted from peripheral blood to examine methylation patterns of specific CpG sites of the *BDNF* promoter (CpG1, CpG2, CpG3, and CpG4) in individuals with MDD compared with unaffected control subjects (Choi et al. 2015). Participants in the study also underwent MRI of the brain, including a diffusion tensor imaging sequence to evaluate and compare white matter integrity. Results showed an inverse correlation between the methylation status of the *BDNF* promoter, specifically at CpG4, and white matter integrity of the right corona radiata, a component of both emotional and cognitive control networks involved in the pathophysiology of MDD. This finding lends support to the idea that a regional BDNF deficit related to DNA hypermethylation could induce neuronal dysfunction in MDD.

Individuals who experience suicidal ideation may carry their own unique epigenetic marks. Over the course of one treatment study, higher *BDNF* methylation levels were found in adults with previous suicide attempt, suicidal ideation during treatment with antidepressants, and suicidal ideation at the last treatment session (Kang et al. 2013). Data from the geriatric population have also demonstrated an association between suicidal ideation at baseline and hypermethylation of the *BDNF* promoter, specifically at CpG5, CpG7, CpG8, and CpG9; furthermore, increased suicidal ideation at 2-year follow-up was tied to hypermethylation specifically at CpG9 (Kim et al. 2014). Hypermethylation of the *TrkB* promoter region has also been positively correlated with depression and suicide over the majority of studies, with the exception of one focusing on promoter methylation in samples taken from Wernicke's area, suggesting this pattern may not be consistent globally across various brain regions (Lockwood et al. 2015).

Several limitations common to many studies examining *BDNF* methylation in MDD should be kept in mind when approaching new research on the topic. First, although some studies have found examples in which DNA methylation of genes in blood cells is associated with that of neural tissue, the findings are both gene and tissue specific, which raises the question of how precisely peripheral blood samples reflect samples taken directly from nervous tissue (see Bakulski et al. [2016] for a review). Second, the methylation status of singular CpG islands or only a few specific sites may provide an incomplete depiction of the methylation status across the entire gene and its promoter regions, as there is no clear consensus on the number of CpG loci required to perform a robust analysis. Third, the functional status of *BDNF* in terms of mRNA expression is not always investigated, meaning there is no verification that increased methylation affects gene expression under the specific conditions of the particular study. Fourth, other factors that may affect *BDNF* methylation status—such as adverse childhood experiences, other forms of psychosocial stressors (see Chapter 4, "Epigenetics of Childhood Trauma and Resilience"), and smoking (see Chapter 5, "Epigenetics of Lifestyle and Aging")—are not always controlled for in study designs. Finally, whether an individual is taking antidepressant medications may affect methylation status, so controls for this variable should also be included in study designs when possible.

Other Epigenetic Contributions to Depression

FKBP5 and Depression

Along with *BDNF*, other genes implicated in the development of MDD have been identified. Studies have shown an association between impaired glucocorticoid signaling, adverse experiences coupled with chronic stress, and development of MDD. This topic is more extensively covered in Chapter 4, "Epigenetics of Childhood Trauma and Resilience", but some associations are worth mentioning here. The **hypothalamic-pituitary-adrenal axis (HPA axis)**, which regulates the **stress response**, is controlled by various genes. Epigenetic factors and variants in these genes contribute to vulnerability to stress-induced depressive pathology. One crucial gene regulator of the axis encodes **FK506 binding protein 51 (FKBP5)** (also named FKBP prolyl isomerase 5). FKBP5 is a co-chaperone of the **glucocorticoid receptor** complex, meaning its role is to assist chaperones—macromolecules that help in conformational folding or unfolding of protein molecules—thus partly regulating glucocorticoid receptor activity in response to chronic stress. The FKBP5 protein inhibits glucocorticoid receptor signaling and can alter glucocorticoid signaling pathway sensitivity. FKBP5 hampers the interaction between the intracellular glucocorticoid receptor and glucocorticoids, thereby impeding intracellular translocation to the nucleus for completion of the signal pathway. In so doing, FKBP5 provides a negative feedback loop of the glucocorticoid signal pathway. The activity and expression of *FKBP5* are influenced by SNPs, the binding of the glucocorticoid receptors to other elements, stressors, and epigenetic modifications. With regard to epigenetic modifications, histone H3 lysine 4 trimethylation (H3K4me3), lysine 27 acetylation (H3K27ac), and lysine 36 trimethylation (H3K36me3)—all of which are hallmarks for expression—are crucial components for this process to function sufficiently (Zannas et al. 2016). Aberrant FKBP5, arising from disruption of any of these pathways, may therefore influence dysregulation of the stress response and is considered a risk factor for developing depression and other affective or anxiety disorders (Binder 2009).

Serotonin Transporter Gene and Depression

The serotonin transporter (SERT; also known as 5-hydroxytryptamine transporter [5-HTT]), which allows reuptake of serotonin into presynaptic neurons, is encoded by the **solute carrier family 6 member 4 (SLC6A4)** gene. The receptor plays a crucial role in the regulation of emotion, affect, and behavior. Variation in the gene and the protein encoded by this gene may alter serotonergic neurotransmission, leading to various emotional and behavioral manifestations. In addition to genetic polymorphisms, regulation of its expression is important in the development of psychopathology. Epigenetic regulation, specifically DNA methylation, of *SLC6A4* has been shown to play a crucial role in its expression. Among studies analyzing DNA methylation of *SLC6A4*, the majority demonstrate increased DNA methylation in individuals with depression (see Chen et al. [2017] for a review). Inconsistencies in this finding across studies may be tied to differences in tissues sampled, depressive phenotypes, or variation in the method of analysis. Regardless, the majority of evidence indicates a trend of increased *SLC6A4* DNA methylation in patients with depression.

Findings From Microarrays

Microarray studies profiling DNA methylation across the genome have identified further regions that may contribute to MDD. In addition, microarray studies offer new perspectives in the etiology of MDD involving multiplex regions of differing DNA methylation. At the time of this writing, there are only a small number of robust works beyond pilot studies.

In a twin study, depression was associated with variation in DNA methylation around regions encoding proteins that play a role in inflammation, including peroxisome proliferator-activated receptor gamma (PPAR-γ), which affects metabolism and modulates immune and inflammatory responses, and activator protein 1 (AP-1), which encodes a transcription factor involved in response to infections and environmental stress (Malki et al. 2016). Numata et al. (2015) found reduced DNA methylation in unmedicated individuals with MDD relative to unaffected control subjects over points of interest including the glycogen synthase kinase 3β gene (*GSK3B*), among others. *GSK3B* plays a role in neural development and energy metabolism, and dysregulated *GSK3B* has been tied to neurodegenerative diseases and bipolar disorder. High expression of *GSK3B* was previously associated with MDD and may play a role in response to antidepressants and lithium, as well as brain changes occurring with MDD.

Numata et al. (2015) reinforced the mosaic pattern of DNA methylation differences, simultaneously discriminating DNA methylation at 17 points to distinguish individuals with MDD from control subjects. Of note, 5% of these DNA methylation differences were found outside gene bodies or promoter regions. Another microarray study found more robust relationships in MDD when profiling multiple locations at once (with an enrichment analysis) than when examining specific, single loci (Oh et al. 2015). Features related to depression showed associations with differences in DNA methylation over networks of loci relevant to biological system processes including metabolism and synaptic function.

Understanding Treatment Response Through Pharmacoepigenetics

Tools to reliably enhance treatment selection and measure treatment response for those with MDD have been a challenge to perfect. Various basic strategies may be used to improve the precision and personalization of medication treatment planning, including considering comorbid diagnoses and medication side effects or selecting a medication class to target specific MDD subtypes (e.g., monoamine oxidase inhibitors [MAOIs] for MDD with atypical features or tricyclic antidepressants [TCAs] for MDD with melancholic features). Additional agents combined with antidepressants, such as antipsychotics for individuals with MDD with psychotic features, or augmentation agents in the case of treatment-resistant depression may also be used. However, some of these strategies bring challenges, including questionable side effect profiles for TCAs and MAOIs and delays in recovery due to the lengthy treatment optimization processes through failed medication trials. Consequently, the need to advance novel, objective tools—such as the identification of biomarkers—is vital as we seek to enhance diagnostic accuracy and effectively measure treatment response.

The field of epigenetics provides a new opportunity to uncover biomarkers for predicting and measuring response to particular medications and treatment modalities. Research in this overlap of pharmacology and epigenetics (**pharmacoepigenetics**) is in its early stages, but findings thus far have been promising. Some potential epigenetic signatures that may serve as biomarkers of treatment responders in MDD include methylation of the genes discussed above (*BDNF*, *TrkB*, and *SLC6A4*), among others (see Belzeaux et al. [2018] and Duclot and Kabbaj [2015] for reviews). A particular example is DNA methylation levels of *BDNF* promoters, which have been shown to be reliable predictors of response to antidepressant treatment. In cases of adults with MDD, lower levels of *BDNF* promoter methylation may be linked to better antidepressant treatment outcomes; higher *BDNF* promoter methylation has been tied to both suicidal ideation throughout the course of treatment and poor treatment outcomes overall (Kang et al. 2013). Histone characteristics including methylation have also emerged as potential biomarkers: for example, in human postmortem studies, use of antidepressants has been found to increase *BDNF* expression in the prefrontal cortex, which was tied to decreased levels of methylated H3K27 at *BDNF* promoter 4 (Chen et al. 2011).

The enzymes involved in deacetylation and methylation more globally, including histone deacetylase (HDAC) and DNA methyltransferase (DNMT), facilitate epigenetic changes and are therefore being considered for their role in treatment response and potential for providing a therapeutic effect. HDAC enzymes have various subtypes and isoforms, and it has been observed that individuals actively experiencing depression may express specific subtypes at different levels than individuals in remission (Belzeaux et al. 2018). Furthermore, several psychotropic medications have been found to themselves yield epigenetic effects, such as valproic acid, which acts as an HDAC inhibitor (Boks et al. 2012). Thus, a better understanding of epigenetic enzyme characterization, including binding sites, function, and relative expression levels of subtypes and isoforms, will provide an indispensable wealth of information for their potential roles as biomarkers for MDD.

Studies examining enzyme phosphorylation are more limited than those examining methylation and acetylation (Hack et al. 2019). However, one study examined the role of DNMT1 in antidepressant treatment response with respect to FKBP5 and BDNF (Gassen et al. 2015). The authors first demonstrated that FKBP5 can prevent phosphorylation of DNMT1. Because phosphorylation of DNMT1 increases the molecule's activity and stability, preventing phosphorylation leads to a reduction of methylation of the genome, including that of *BDNF*, in turn promoting expression. The authors then took samples of peripheral blood mononuclear cells before and after a 6-week treatment course with antidepressants. Change in DNMT1 phosphorylation over that time period was correlated with rated depressive symptom reduction, such that greater decreases in phosphorylation were related to greater improvements in depressive symptoms. In tandem, the authors controlled for environmental factors and isolated the effects of antidepressants on these proteins by treating the same patients' blood cells taken at the initial visit with paroxetine ex vivo (outside the patient's body, in the laboratory). The reduction in DNMT1 phosphorylation in the laboratory setting remained correlated with improvement in depressive symptoms experienced by the individual. Therefore, whether administered therapeutically in vivo or to the blood ex vivo, treatment with antidepressants may lead to changes in DNMT1 functioning to a degree predictive of that individual's treatment response. Similarly, individuals who did not show much clinical response to antidepressant treatment exhibited higher phosphorylation of DNMT1 both in blood cells taken after treatment in vivo and in blood cells treated ex vivo with paroxetine. Concurrently, increased *BDNF* expression was positively correlated with FKBP5 levels in both in vivo and ex vivo samples. Results therefore reveal that the effects of antidepressant medication may be modulated by FKBP5 through a downregulating effect on the epigenetic machinery DNMT1, ultimately increasing expression of *BDNF*, suggesting the potential utility of DNMT1 phosphorylation levels serving as a biomarker for predicting antidepressant treatment response.

HDAC inhibitors could potentially decrease the deacetylation process, providing an antidepressant effect. One compound that has been found to yield antidepressant effects is **sodium butyrate**, which is available through dietary sources and may be synthesized in the body. Sodium butyrate acts as an HDAC inhibitor with additional enzymatic effects that lead to downstream DNA demethylation. In one rodent study, administration of sodium butyrate was found to produce antidepressant effects while increasing enzymatic activity that downregulated *Bdnf* methylation in the prefrontal cortex, increasing expression (Wei et al. 2014). Another compound available through diet and biosynthesis that acts similarly to an HDAC inhibitor is L-**acetylcarnitine (LAC)**, which has been found to have antidepressant effects as well. Through epigenetic regulation of a particular glutamate receptor, LAC has been shown to yield quick and lasting improvement in depressive symptoms in rodents with genetic vulnerability or exposure to toxic stress (Nasca et al. 2013). The possible mechanism for this is understood to involve increasing levels of acetylated H3K27 binding to the promoters of both the glutamate receptor gene and *Bdnf* in neural tissue, increasing expression of both.

Expanding the scope from drug administration to other medical interventions, there is limited but promising evidence regarding potential epigenetic signatures of response to electroconvulsive therapy (ECT) (Feng and Youssef 2020). Changes in DNA methylation between time points before and after a course of ECT have been revealed to correlate with treatment response (Sirignano et al. 2021). One CpG site notable for its association with a robust treatment response is associated with *TNKS*, which encodes a protein with a variety of cellular functions, including telomere length regulation, vesicle transportation, spindle assembly, and Wnt signal transduction pathway, and has been associated with affective disorders. *FKBP5* also shows changes in DNA methylation patterns related to improvement in depressive symptoms following ECT. Other studies have found additional locations of interest regarding ECT response in individuals with treatment-resistant depression, in particular elevated promoter DNA methylation of P11, a calcium-binding protein relevant to depression and antidepressant effects (Neyazi et al. 2018; Svenningsson et al. 2013). Although not yet ready for clinical application, pharmacoepigenetics has already yielded noteworthy findings in the field of psychiatry and continues to expand the horizon for monitoring and predicting treatment response.

Conclusion

Despite a long history of study, MDD remains difficult to treat and is among the most prevalent psychiatric disorders. Advances improving our understanding of the disorder and its treatment have arisen from the application of epigenetics to the field of psychiatry. Highlighted in this chapter is the role that BDNF may play in the etiology of MDD. The epigenetic regulation of *BDNF* has been relatively well studied, providing information regarding the development of MDD, its pathophysiology, and its response to treatment. As with other genes, expression of *BDNF* is associated with epigenetic markings such as DNA methylation and histone methylation/acetylation. The epigenetic marks give information (i.e., act as a biomarker) for MDD symptoms and also provide a potential mechanism for development of pathology in MDD, along with genetic predispositions and environmental exposure to elicit symptom expression. In addition to BDNF, factors involved in epigenetic regulation within MDD include the serotonin receptor and components of glucocorticoid receptor functioning. Therefore, whether conceptualizing MDD through the monoamine hypothesis, the BDNF hypothesis, or the stress response, epigenetic mechanisms play a role in its etiology and thus its treatment. As will be discussed in the upcoming chapters, the applications of epigenetics in psychiatry go far beyond understanding depression. As the field of epigenetics continues to grow, its potential impacts on the field of psychiatry will likewise expand.

KEY POINTS

- The relationship between environmental factors, such as stress, and the development of depression and other disorders may be driven in part by effects on brain-derived neurotrophic factor (BDNF). BDNF is a neuronal growth factor that stimulates neuronal development, plasticity, synaptogenesis, and long-term potentiation.

- With 11 exons and 9 promoters, the gene encoding BDNF can be transcribed into a variety of mRNA transcripts, allowing for regulation based on cell type, tissue region, and activity level. Despite numerous possible mRNA sequences, the same BDNF precursor protein is translated, which is ultimately cleaved before becoming the mature, functional BDNF protein. Some variability in BDNF structure is possible, though, from single-nucleotide polymorphisms (SNPs) creating different allele forms. Such differences in BDNF structure have been tied to susceptibility to pathology.

- Research on animal models has demonstrated that increasing BDNF endogenously or exogenously can improve or reverse the depressive and cognitive symptoms associated with excessive environmental stress. Such toxic stress can downregulate *BDNF* expression through DNA methylation changes and histone modification.

- Research in clinical populations has replicated findings from research in animal models, in which depressive symptoms are associated with BDNF functioning, tied to *BDNF* promoter methylation status. Major depressive disorder (MDD) specifically has been linked to hypermethylation of the *BDNF* promoter region longitudinally. Particular sites and patterns of hypermethylation in the same promoter region also emerge as predictors of suicidal ideation in depression.

- FK506 binding protein 51 (FKBP5) is a co-chaperone of the glucocorticoid receptor complex, playing an inhibitory role, ultimately contributing to a negative feedback loop of the glucocorticoid signal pathway. Epigenetic effects on FKBP5 expression, evoked by significant environmental stressors, have been linked to increased risk of developing depression and other mood and anxiety disorders. Evidence supports methylation and acetylation at particular histone sites as one mechanism of this epigenetic effect.

- The serotonin transporter (SERT) has also been linked to the depressive phenotype; in particular, some epigenetic modifications correlate with depression status. The majority of studies have indicated a relationship between DNA hypermethylation of *SLC6A4* and depression.

- Pharmacoepigenetics—the application of epigenetics to understanding medical treatment response—provides an avenue for understanding and possibly predicting treatment response. Research thus far has demonstrated the role of DNA methylation and histone modification of *BDNF* and other genes in predicting antidepressant treatment response. Furthermore, the enzymes that drive epigenetic mechanisms, including histone deacetylase (HDAC) and DNA methyltransferase (DNMT), appear to play a role in anti-depressant treatment response and may even be harnessed for a potential therapeutic effect. Individuals with treatment-resistant depression who respond positively to electroconvulsive therapy (ECT) may also carry their own epigenetic signatures.

Study Questions

1. Which of the following is true regarding the DNA, RNA, and protein structure of brain-derived neurotrophic factor (BDNF)?

    A. *BDNF* has 11 exons with 9 functional tissue-specific promoters, creating a variety of mRNA transcripts, leading to variations in structure of BDNF across tissues.
    B. Varieties of mRNA transcripts of *BDNF* are expressed similarly and randomly across cell types and regions, but the BDNF protein structure does not vary within an individual.
    C. Varieties of mRNA transcripts of *BDNF* are typically specific to cell type, region, and activity; BDNF structure may vary between individuals.
    D. Varieties of mRNA transcripts of *BDNF* are typically specific to cell type, region, and activity, without BDNF structure varying between individuals.

    Best answer: C

    Explanation: The human gene *BDNF* has 11 exons with 9 functional tissue-specific promoters. As a result, a wide variety of mRNA transcripts are created. The transcription of *BDNF* can be regulated in a tissue- and activity-specific manner based on the numerous exons and promoters, meaning that particular mRNA transcripts are typically seen in cells of the same type and region (contradicting answer B). Despite this variety of mRNA transcripts, they all encode the same protein precursor (if from the same allele), which is cleaved through a process ultimately yielding BDNF (unlike answer A). BDNF protein structure is expected to be consistent; however, due to single-nucleotide polymorphisms (SNPs), BDNF structure may vary between individuals, or one individual may express two different BDNF structures if heterozygous (contradicting answer D).

2.   Which of the following epigenetic changes has been implicated in the development of major depressive disorder (MDD)?

A. *BDNF* DNA demethylation
B. *BDNF* SNPs
C. Histone H3 lysine 4 trimethylation (H3K4me3), lysine 27 acetylation (H3K27ac), and lysine 36 trimethylation (H3K36me3)
D. *BDNF* DNA methylation

Best answer: D

Explanation: It has been studied and noted that methylation at various cytosine-[phosphate]-guanine dinucleotide (CpG) sites of the *BDNF* promoter region has been implicated in the development of MDD and other depressive phenotypes including suicidality. Epigenetic studies of *BDNF* typically demonstrate that individuals with MDD carry relatively high levels of methylation (not demethylation as in answer A) in the promoter region of this gene, understood to be associated with lower expression of *BDNF* and subsequent neurological effects, with changes to cognitive and affective regulation. Generally, methylation is a hallmark for gene repression, and demethylation, a hallmark for gene expression. There is deviation from this general notion, however. For example, histone H3 lysine 4 trimethylation (H3K4me3), lysine 27 acetylation (H3K27ac), and lysine 36 trimethylation (H3K36me3) have notable effects on gene expression of *FKBP5*, which is protective of the hypothalamic-pituitary-adrenal (HPA) axis and would not be associated with the development of MDD (answer C). SNPs (answer B) are genetic changes, not epigenetic modifications.

3.   According to a majority of the evidence, individuals with MDD show

A. Increased DNA methylation of the serotonin transporter (*SLC6A4*) gene promoter
B. Decreased DNA methylation of the tropomyosin receptor kinase B (*TrkB*) gene promoter
C. Increased histone acetyltransferase (HAT) activity
D. Decreased DNA methyltransferase (DNMT) activity

Best answer: A

MDD has been associated with decreased expression of relevant genes, including *BDNF*, *SLC6A4*, and *TrkB*. Often, increased methylation of a promoter region is associated with decreased expression of the gene, as is the case with *SLC6A4*. TrkB is a major BDNF receptor, and hypermethylation of the *TrkB* promoter region (associated with decreased expression) has been positively correlated with depression and suicide over many studies (answer B). DNMT and HAT are enzymes crucial to methylation and acetylation, respectively. DNMT facilitates the addition of a methyl group to the cytosine of a CpG dinucleotide; therefore, decreased activity of DNMT is typically associated with decreased DNA methylation (answer D). HAT facilitates the addition of an acetyl group to lysine of histones, which, in general, lets DNA become more accessible to transcription, increasing expression (answer C).

4.   Which of the following is true regarding neuropsychiatric epigenetics research using peripheral blood samples from clinical populations?

     A. DNA methylation patterns are nearly identical across tissues, so samples taken from peripheral blood cells are practically equivalent to those taken from brain tissue.

     B. DNA methylation patterns in peripheral blood cells have shown an association with that of neural tissue in some studies, but this is gene and tissue specific.

     C. DNA methylation patterns in peripheral blood cells are useful only when studying proteins that cross the blood–brain barrier.

     D. DNA methylation patterns in peripheral blood cells do not approximate those of neural tissue and therefore do not have utility in the clinical research setting.

Best answer: B

Explanation: A consideration when approaching clinical research is the tissue source of the DNA, particularly whether it was taken from peripheral blood or neural tissue. Each tissue source brings both limitations and advantages for research. Studies using neurological tissue samples provide an opportunity to study the mechanisms underlying pathology but require postmortem samples, creating limitations to data available for phenotyping, restricting studies to small sample sizes, and obviating longitudinal follow-up. Studies using samples from peripheral blood do not face these same limitations, but they raise the question of how closely the methylation patterns of DNA in blood approximate those of specific brain structures, as these are not automatically equivalent (contradicting answer A). Some studies have demonstrated an association in particular instances where DNA methylation patterns taken from peripheral blood strongly correlate with target neural structures, demonstrating that there is merit to this technique (negating answer D), but this is gene and tissue specific (answer C is too narrow). Therefore, cross-tissue studies are necessary to demonstrate the validity of the technique when practical, to demonstrate that peripheral blood may serve as a proxy for the brain given the particular gene and tissues being studied.

References

Bakulski KM, Halladay A, Hu VW, et al: Epigenetic research in neuropsychiatric disorders: the "tissue issue." Curr Behav Neurosci Rep 3(3):264–274, 2016 28093577

Belzeaux R, Lin R, Ju C, et al: Transcriptomic and epigenomic biomarkers of antidepressant response. J Affect Disord 233:36–44, 2018 28918100

Binder EB: The role of FKBP5, a co-chaperone of the glucocorticoid receptor in the pathogenesis and therapy of affective and anxiety disorders. Psychoneuroendocrinology 34(Suppl 1):S186–S195, 2009 19560279

Boks MP, de Jong NM, Kas MJ, et al: Current status and future prospects for epigenetic psychopharmacology. Epigenetics 7(1):20–28, 2012 22207355

Cattaneo A, Cattane N, Begni V, et al: The human BDNF gene: peripheral gene expression and protein levels as biomarkers for psychiatric disorders. Transl Psychiatry 6(11):e958, 2016 27874848

Chen D, Meng L, Pei F, et al: A review of DNA methylation in depression. J Clin Neurosci 43:39–46, 2017 28645747

Chen ES, Ernst C, Turecki G: The epigenetic effects of antidepressant treatment on human prefrontal cortex BDNF expression. Int J Neuropsychopharmacol 14(3):427–429, 2011 21134314

Chen KW, Chen L: Epigenetic regulation of BDNF gene during development and diseases. Int J Mol Sci 18(3):571, 2017 28272318

Choi S, Han KM, Won E, et al: Association of brain-derived neurotrophic factor DNA methylation and reduced white matter integrity in the anterior corona radiata in major depression. J Affect Disord 172:74–80, 2015 25451398

Dell'Osso B, D'Addario C, Carlotta Palazzo M, et al: Epigenetic modulation of BDNF gene: differences in DNA methylation between unipolar and bipolar patients. J Affect Disord 166:330–333, 2014 25012449

Duclot F, Kabbaj M: Epigenetic mechanisms underlying the role of brain-derived neurotrophic factor in depression and response to antidepressants. J Exp Biol 218(Pt 1):21–31, 2015 25568448

Duman RS, Heninger GR, Nestler EJ: A molecular and cellular theory of depression. Arch Gen Psychiatry 54(7):597–606, 1997 9236543

Feng T, Youssef NA: Can epigenetic biomarkers lead us to precision medicine in predicting treatment response and remission for patients being considered for ECT? Psychiatry Res 284:112659, 2020 31703983

Gassen NC, Fries GR, Zannas AS, et al: Chaperoning epigenetics: FKBP51 decreases the activity of DNMT1 and mediates epigenetic effects of the antidepressant paroxetine. Sci Signal 8(404):ra119, 2015 26602018

Hack LM, Fries GR, Eyre HA, et al: Moving pharmacoepigenetics tools for depression toward clinical use. J Affect Disord 249:336–346, 2019 30802699

Hing B, Sathyaputri L, Potash JB: A comprehensive review of genetic and epigenetic mechanisms that regulate BDNF expression and function with relevance to major depressive disorder. Am J Med Genet B Neuropsychiatr Genet 177(2):143–167, 2018 29243873

Ignácio ZM, Réus GZ, Abelaira HM, Quevedo J: Epigenetic and epistatic interactions between serotonin transporter and brain-derived neurotrophic factor genetic polymorphism: insights in depression. Neuroscience 275:455–468, 2014 24972302

Kang HJ, Kim JM, Lee JY, et al: BDNF promoter methylation and suicidal behavior in depressive patients. J Affect Disord 151(2):679–685, 2013 23992681

Kang HJ, Kim JM, Kim SY, et al: A longitudinal study of BDNF promoter methylation and depression in breast cancer. Psychiatry Investig 12(4):523–531, 2015 26508964

Kim JM, Kang HJ, Bae KY, et al: Association of BDNF promoter methylation and genotype with suicidal ideation in elderly Koreans. Am J Geriatr Psychiatry 22(10):989–996, 2014 24731781

Lockwood LE, Su S, Youssef NA: The role of epigenetics in depression and suicide: a platform for gene-environment interactions. Psychiatry Res 228(3):235–242, 2015 26163724

Malki K, Koritskaya E, Harris F, et al: Epigenetic differences in monozygotic twins discordant for major depressive disorder. Translat Psychiatr 6(6):e839, 2016

Nagahara AH, Tuszynski MH: Potential therapeutic uses of BDNF in neurological and psychiatric disorders. Nat Rev Drug Discov 10(3):209–219, 2011 21358740

Nasca C, Xenos D, Barone Y, et al: L-acetylcarnitine causes rapid antidepressant effects through the epigenetic induction of mGlu2 receptors. Proc Natl Acad Sci USA 110(12):4804–4809, 2013

Neyazi A, Theilmann W, Brandt C, et al: P11 promoter methylation predicts the antidepressant effect of electroconvulsive therapy. Transl Psychiatry 8(1):25, 2018 29353887

Numata S, Ishii K, Tajima A, et al: Blood diagnostic biomarkers for major depressive disorder using multiplex DNA methylation profiles: discovery and validation. Epigenet 10(2):135–141, 2015

Oh G, Wang SC, Pal M, et al: DNA modification study of major depressive disorder: beyond locus-by-locus comparisons. Biol Psychiatr 77(3):246–255, 2015

Pruunsild P, Kazantseva A, Aid T, et al: Dissecting the human BDNF locus: bi-directional transcription, complex splicing, and multiple promoters. Genomics 90(3):397–406, 2007 17629449

Roth TL, Lubin FD, Funk AJ, Sweatt JD: Lasting epigenetic influence of early life adversity on the BDNF gene. Biol Psychiatry 65(9):760–769, 2009 19150054

Roy B, Shelton RC, Dwivedi Y: DNA methylation and expression of stress related genes in PBMC of MDD patients with and without serious suicidal ideation. J Psychiatr Res 89:115–124, 2017 28246044

Sirignano L, Frank J, Kranaster L, et al: Methylome-wide change associated with response to electroconvulsive therapy in depressed patients. Transl Psychiatry 11(1):347, 2021 34091594

Svenningsson P, Kim Y, Warner-Schmidt J, et al: p11 and its role in depression and therapeutic responses to antidepressants. Nat Rev Neurosci 14(10):673–680, 2013 24002251

Uchida S, Yamagata H, Seki T, Watanabe Y: Epigenetic mechanisms of major depression: Targeting neuronal plasticity. Psychiatry Clin Neurosci 72(4):212–227, 2018 29154458

Wei Y, Melas PA, Wegener G, et al: Antidepressant-like effect of sodium butyrate is associated with an increase in TET1 and in 5-hydroxymethylation levels in the Bdnf gene. Int J Neuropsychopharmacol 18(2):pyu032, 2014 25618518

Zannas AS, Wiechmann T, Gassen NC, Binder EB: Gene-stress-epigenetic regulation of FKBP5: clinical and translational implications. Neuropsychopharmacology 41(1):261–274, 2016 26250598

Epigenetics in Neurodevelopmental and Neurodegenerative Disorders

Kyle J. Rutledge, D.O., Ph.D.
Onoriode Edeh, M.D.

Within the field of psychiatry, a thorough discussion of epigenetics would be incomplete if certain neurodevelopmental and neurodegenerative disorders were not included. We include this list of disorders (which is not exhaustive) on the basis of what information is available currently and could lead to a better understanding of epigenetics in psychiatry. These neurodevelopmental disorders highlight the principles of epigenetics, and in so doing, increase understanding of the developmental etiology of these disorders.

As described in Chapter 1, "Overview of Genetic and Epigenetic Mechanisms," three methods have been used historically to study DNA methylation, although the science continues to develop. One method examines methylation patterns globally and nonspecifically, looking at relative percentages of cytosine methylation across regions, without specifically denoting where these methylated bases are located. Another is the theory-driven single-gene or candidate-gene approach, in which a single target gene is identified a priori and isolated, and cytosine methylation status is examined along relevant regions such as CpG islands. The third method, the most recent and advanced, is more data driven and looks at genome-wide methylation patterns, producing gene sequences and denoting which specific cytosine bases are methylated.

Historically, single-gene approaches have been emphasized in the field of psychiatry, but as research has progressed, the heritable components of these disorders have been revealed to be more and more complex. It is uncommon for a psychiatric illness to be well explained by a single gene (with standout exceptions being Huntington's disease and fragile X syndrome). The complexity is in part due to **polygenic inheritance** patterns, in which a pattern of multiple genes is passed along to the next generation. De novo mutations, which occur spontaneously during DNA replication and are not shared with either parent, are not uncommon. Routinely found as more genetic and epigenetic data are collected are **variants of uncertain significance**: a variant is found at a particular locus, but it is unclear whether the difference corresponds to a clinically significant outcome. Further, many genes are **pleiotropic**, meaning that variations in a single gene and its expression yield multiple phenotypic traits. Epigenetics, of course, adds further layers of complexity to the etiology of these disorders. Therefore, studies are shifting their research methods toward genomewide and epigenomewide association studies.

With the exception of fetal alcohol syndrome, the disorders described in this chapter have been demonstrated as having clear genetic underpinnings (i.e., changes to the gene sequence). Important epigenetic mechanisms and regulatory processes are also involved in each disorder. First, we discuss schizophrenia, which in recent decades has become understood as a neurodevelopmental disorder. Next, we explore autism spectrum disorder, followed by Rett syndrome, in which a genetic mutation leads to dysregulation of the body's epigenetic machinery. Additional syndromes—Prader-Willi and Angelman—are most commonly associated with gene mutations, with different pathologies emerging owing to the epigenetic processes of imprinting. The effects of **trinucleotide repeat expansions** in the chromosomes in fragile X syndrome and Huntington's disease have also been associated with measurable epigenetic effects that lead to development of pathology.

Schizophrenia

Psychotic disorders including **schizophrenia** attract significant attention in health care. Despite low prevalence relative to other psychiatric diagnoses, schizophrenia carries a significant burden for patients, families, and social/economic resources (Chong et al. 2016). DSM-5-TR diagnostic criteria (American Psychiatric Association 2022) include a variety of positive (e.g., hallucinations, delusions) and negative (e.g., prosody of speech, social withdrawal, anhedonia) symptoms, indicating the clinical heterogeneity of the disorder. Similarly, biological correlates have been found to be rather broad, both at the neurotransmitter level (involving much more than dopamine dysregulation [Yang and Tsai 2017]) and at the neuroanatomic level (with widespread reductions in total brain volume, including both gray and white matter [Woodward and Heckers 2015]). Despite these broad characterizations at the clinical and neurobiological levels, schizophrenia has a high heritability rate of 79%–83% (similar to those of other psychotic disorders) and a relatively low concordance rate of 0.33 in monozygotic twins and 0.07 in dizygotic twins, highlighting the disorder's heterogeneity and the contributions of environmental factors in disease expression (Hilker et al. 2018).

Genetic research has reliably shown that schizophrenia is not explained by individual genes, but rather is tied to variants at multiple gene sites, some common with low **penetrance** and others uncommon with high penetrance (Avramopoulos 2018). It has been hypothesized that because individuals with schizophrenia are less likely to have offspring than the general population, negative selection exists for risk alleles. Thus the more common alleles that remain in the gene pool carry low contributions to risk of developing the disorder. More than 100 genetic loci have been found to be significant for schizophrenia, including independent ties to dopaminergic, glutamatergic, and immunological pathways (Ripke et al. 2014). In this way, schizophrenia exemplifies the utility of genomewide studies that explore variance at multiple sites across the genome. Further, study of the epigenetics of schizophrenia necessitates an epigenomewide approach.

It is worth noting that patterns have emerged with **copy number variants (CNVs)**, in which portions of the chromosome are deleted or duplicated, and which may be de novo or inherited. A notable example is velocardiofacial syndrome (or DiGeorge syndrome), which is caused by a deletion of chromosomal band 22q11.2, leading to palatal, cardiac, and facial effects (as the name indicates) in addition to learning difficulties, behavior dysregulation, and chronic psychosis later in life. Outside that region, increased levels of CNVs have been found globally in individuals with schizophrenia, including in regions previously tied to neurobehavioral and synaptic function (Marshall et al. 2017). Because several locations may be tied to development of psychosis, efforts are underway to adopt microarrays including known CNVs for schizophrenia to aid in counseling and treatment of individuals in the clinical setting (Chen et al. 2021).

Beyond heredity and gene variant effects, environmental risk factors have been found to influence etiology. Perinatal exposures may contribute to the development of schizophrenia: higher rates are associated with obstetric complications and maternal malnutrition and illness. In fact, individuals born in winter or spring months carry an increased risk of developing schizophrenia (Torrey et al. 1977). Cannabis use is dose-dependently connected with the risk of developing schizophrenia (Marconi et al. 2016). Tobacco use also strongly correlates with schizophrenia, with a questionable direction of causality. Additional risk factors include childhood trauma, lower education level, and elevated stress (Fusar-Poli et al. 2017). There is some evidence that these factors impart risk through epigenetic mechanisms (Richetto and Meyer 2021; Smigielski et al. 2020).

Nonspecific global DNA methylation measures have shown mixed results depending on source tissue (blood vs. brain): some studies have correlated disease expression with higher global DNA methylation patterns, and others, with lower global DNA methylation (Smigielski et al. 2020). Candidate gene studies have found relationships between schizophrenia development and DNA methylation of genes tied to the dopaminergic, serotonergic, and GABAergic systems (Roth et al. 2009). With respect to dopamine, the **catechol-*O*-methyltransferase (*COMT*)** gene, which is located within 22q11 (the same region affected in velocardiofacial syndrome) and encodes an enzyme that breaks down catecholamines, has polymorphisms that can increase risk of schizophrenia; furthermore, there is evidence that DNA methylation differences affect *COMT* expression in some individuals with the disorder. Some (albeit inconsistent) evidence suggests that methylation of the serotonin 2A receptor gene (*HTR2A*) promoter may also be dysregulated, with subsequent effects on receptor expression in the schizophrenia brain. In the γ-**aminobutyric acid (GABA)** system, candidate gene approaches have investigated **glutamate decarboxylase 1 (*GAD1*)** and **reelin (*RELN*)** gene regulatory regions. Reelin, which is involved in the regulatory function of neurons with effects on migration and synaptic plasticity, is expressed by types of neurodevelopmentally relevant GABAergic neurons, and expression has been found to be reduced in schizophrenia. *GAD1* synthesizes GABA from glutamate and has also been found to be differentially expressed in schizophrenia. Studies have indicated disruption of DNA methylation in the regulatory regions of both *RELN* and *GAD1*, contributing to downregulated expression.

Genomewide methylation studies have shown patterns of DNA methylation that are less replicable, suggesting that patterns are individualized for cases of schizophrenia (Smigielski et al. 2020). This consistent finding of a variety of DNA methylation patterns across the genome of people meeting diagnostic criteria for schizophrenia parallels genetic studies in which the disorder stems from a variety of common variants with low penetrance and rare variants with high penetrance across the genome. This theme also reflects the disorder's heterogeneity in clinical manifestations. The results of these studies are far reaching, continuously updated, and too complex to be reviewed here; some regions have remained relevant, including *COMT* and *RELN*, as well as other sites showing themes of effects on metabolic/mitochondrial and inflammatory processes. Furthermore, pharmacoepigenetic studies have shown that DNA methylation patterns may predict antipsychotic treatment response and may change longitudinally with antipsychotic treatment (Lisoway et al. 2021).

Beyond epigenetic variance at specific sites, problems with epigenetic machinery may lead to schizophrenia and developmental delay. Development of schizophrenia has been tied to rare genetic variants leading to loss of function of *SETD1A*, encoding a histone methyltransferase specifically targeting H3K4 (Singh et al. 2016). This rare but substantial effect suggests that proper regulation of methylation of histones at H3K4 is instrumental to typical neurodevelopment, and that dysregulation may lead to downstream effects including schizophrenia. H3 has been further showcased as a site for epigenetic modification in schizophrenia, as the disorder has been tied to increases in methylation of H3K9 (Chase et al. 2013) and phosphorylation of H3K10 (Sharma et al. 2015).

The multifactorial development and clinical presentation of schizophrenia parallel the heterogeneity of genetic and epigenetic contributions to the disorder. Its complex etiology demonstrates how single-gene approaches may fall short in characterizing many psychiatric disorders. Genome- and epigenomewide studies, including microarrays, with their capacity for uncovering novel loci, multiple pathways, and patterns of genetic and epigenetic variations, are therefore proliferating.

Autism Spectrum Disorder

Autism spectrum disorder (ASD) is another neurodevelopmental disorder with a complex etiology. ASD emerges in early childhood, with features including deficient social-emotional reciprocity, abnormal communication, restrictive behaviors, and fixed interests. Some ASD cases may be tied to other conditions with known genetic causes, as in the case of fragile X syndrome or Rett syndrome, discussed later in this chapter. However, as with schizophrenia, most cases seem to rise from more complicated roots, through heritable and de novo genetic vulnerabilities interacting with environmental factors. Because of these multigene predispositions, single-gene approaches to understanding the disorder have provided a limited picture, with genetic and epigenetic research turning toward genome- and epigenomewide measures including microarrays.

Genomewide studies have identified numerous risk loci containing polymorphisms associated with development of ASD, many of which overlap with development of schizophrenia (The Psychiatric Genomics Consortium 2017). As with schizophrenia, each gene variant explains only a small portion (<1%) of cases, and the majority of cases of ASD are not tied to a specific genetic abnormality. However, many risk loci are associated with neurodevelopment and broad epigenetic regulation, affecting brain development. As knowledge of these loci continues to expand, information is tracked using databases such as the **Simons Foundation Autism Research Initiative (SFARI Gene)** database, which is frequently updated and available to researchers (Abrahams et al. 2013). Also, given the lack of robust single-gene contributions to ASD, researchers taking genomewide approaches also perform **gene set enrichment analysis (GSEA)** (or network enrichment analysis as described in Chapter 1, "Overview of Genetic and Epigenetic Mechanisms"), in which related parts of the genome (having similar biological function, genome position, or other statistical association) are investigated in a sample for enrichment or overrepresentation of CpG sites, with methylation differences emerging in the data.

One environmental factor that has been linked to preventing the development of ASD is in utero folic acid supplementation, which may act through folate's key role in the methylation of DNA. Higher folic acid intake before conception and through the first month of gestation—a period of significant DNA demethylation and remethylation for offspring—has been linked to a lower incidence of ASD (see Ciernia and LaSalle [2016] for a review). This association may be related to the relationship between increased folic acid intake and DNA methylation patterns in sites key to development across human and animal studies. Other risk factors associated with DNA methylation and neurodevelopmental consequences include in utero exposure to nicotine, cannabis, alcohol, heavy metals, and air pollutants.

High-throughput methods, which have the power to uncover novel patterns and regions of interest, have not found consistent patterns of

DNA methylation across ASD (Andrews et al. 2018); however, distinct patterns have emerged for subsets of individuals with ASD. Some distinct patterns of DNA methylation are based on particular genetic risk factors. In a small study including individuals with ASD, those who carried 16p11.2 deletions showed specific patterns of DNA methylation across the genome, differentiating them from individuals carrying risk alleles for *CHD8*, which encodes an epigenetically relevant helicase binding protein that has a regulatory effect on chromatin remodeling, further distinguishing them from others diagnosed with ASD and control subjects (Siu et al. 2019).

In a study using whole-genome bisulfite sequencing of cord blood samples from birth to locate methylated cytosines across the genome, patterns of DNA methylation were distinct in individuals who went on to be diagnosed with ASD (Mordaunt et al. 2020). Identified regions occurred around genes relevant to neurodevelopment, and distinct regions differed between males and females. Another study, which used an Illumina microarray containing 450,000 sites to examine cord blood and placental tissue of children later diagnosed with ASD, again did not find specific sites of DNA methylation changes consistent across ASD cases compared with unaffected control subjects but did find enrichment of CpG sites over ASD risk areas defined by the SFARI Gene database (Bakulski et al. 2021).

Rett Syndrome

Rett syndrome (RTT) is a neurodevelopmental disorder that has received much research attention, particularly with respect to genetic and epigenetic processes. The disorder itself is rare, affecting about one in 10,000 people, but the nuances of its etiology help illuminate many of the genetic and epigenetic processes associated with common neurodevelopmental disorders (see Table 3–1).

RTT almost exclusively affects females, with few exceptions. After 6–18 months of otherwise normal development, symptoms of RTT emerge wherein an individual begins to regress in communication and motor development, losing acquired milestones. As RTT progresses, additional features emerge. Although the disorder primarily impacts the central nervous system, symptoms are found across multiple organ systems. Neurologically, patients demonstrate apraxia, seizures, dysphasia, intellectual disability, and microcephaly. Psychiatrically, patients demonstrate autistic-like behaviors (e.g., stereotypical hand movements and social

Table 3–1.   Clinical insights: assessment and intervention in Rett syndrome

---

Assessment

◆ Although RTT predominantly affects those with two X chromosomes (females), rare cases occur in those with one X and one Y chromosome (males), and they typically have a worse prognosis.

◆ It is essential to gather a thorough family history, searching for other cases of RTT or other potential developmental disorders in the family.

◆ In a patient with developmental delay, rule out more common causes first. If the patient has a developmental delay and no clinical markers toward RTT specifically, perform a chromosomal microarray, then specific metabolic testing, and then fragile X syndrome testing. If no conclusion is reached from these tests, then it is appropriate to test for *MECP2*.

◆ Order an ECG to assess for QTc prolongation, which is relatively more common in those with RTT.

Treatment

◆ No modality or treatment regimen is currently available specifically for RTT. Treatment planning revolves around management of associated conditions.

◆ Genetic counseling is crucial in cases of RTT, and parents need anticipatory guidance.

◆ Coordinate with a multispecialty team including neurology (potential comorbid epilepsy), orthopedics (common issues with bone health, scoliosis), gastroenterology (eating difficulties, constipation), occupational therapy/physical therapy, and nutrition (calcium and vitamin D for bone health).

◆ Individuals with RTT will live into adulthood with ongoing intensive ancillary care needs.

Additional resources

◆ The International Rett Syndrome Foundation provides information for families and pathways for genetic testing.

◆ The Rett Syndrome Research Trust focuses on research but also provides networking opportunities and other resources specific to RTT for families.

Note.   ECG = electrocardiogram; RTT = Rett syndrome.

withdrawal), depression, and self-injurious behavior. Despite the initial pattern of social withdrawal, as individuals with RTT grow older, they become much more social and interactive. Although expressive language remains a challenge, they demonstrate adequate receptive language.

Patients with RTT show lifelong deficits and require ongoing care. In spite of the multiple medical comorbidities with grave prognoses (arrhythmias, risk for aspiration, seizures, etc.), many individuals with RTT live well into adulthood.

Beyond the impact it has on patients and families, RTT is notable for its genetic etiology. The syndrome is often lumped into "epigenetic" disorders, but to be clear, RTT is caused by a single gene mutation. The gene affected, **methyl CpG-binding protein 2 (*MeCP2*)**, encodes a protein that binds to methylated cytosine in cytosine-[phosphate]-guanine (CpG) islands, affecting the regulation of associated genes. MeCP2 itself, therefore, is intimately involved in epigenetic regulation of gene expression. Mutations to *MeCP2* in RTT lead to a loss of function of the protein. Thus RTT is a disorder caused by a gene mutation that leads to organism-wide dysfunction of epigenetic mechanisms.

MeCP2 has further influences on many biological pathways, and at the time of this writing, these pathways and the entire phenotype of RTT are not fully understood. However, MeCP2 appears to be necessary for proliferation and maturation of neural stem cells. Problems with *MeCP2* therefore affect early neurogenesis, neuronal migration, and cortical patterning, leading to disrupted circuits and compromised synaptic plasticity and transmission, as well as changes to glial cells (Feldman et al. 2016; Qiu 2018).

The function of MeCP2 seems primarily to connect portions of DNA to other proteins. To achieve this, the structure of MeCP2 includes a DNA-binding domain that targets methylated bases on the genome, most predominantly cytosine in CpG islands, as the name "methyl CpG-binding protein" indicates. After binding to methylated cytosine, the other binding regions of MeCP2 may interact with additional proteins to create chromosome-protein complexes that may function to affect the epigenetic regulation of gene expression. Although understood to predominantly repress gene transcription, these complexes may also activate transcription of some genes or become involved in facilitating microRNA (miRNA) processing (Horvath and Monteggia 2018; Lyst and Bird 2015).

MeCP2 has been mapped to the X chromosome, where RTT is most often caused by a spontaneous mutation that is not inherited. Because RTT is X-linked, patients are female, with some exceptions (Villard et al. 2000). Generally only one of the two X chromosomes in a female carries the mutation, and the other carries a functional *MeCP2* gene; random X chromosome inactivation means there is a 50% chance that the mutant gene will escape X-inactivation and the functional (wild-type) gene will be silenced. Therefore, approximately half of cells will express the mutant gene, and the other half will express the functional gene (Przanowski et al. 2018).

Not every cell type shows effects. *MeCP2* is naturally expressed differently in different areas of the body, with greater activity in the brain than other organs. Furthermore, the timing of symptom onset—emerging ~6–18 months after a period of normal development—is when the outward effects of this deficiency in epigenetic regulation become apparent enough for clinical detection. Therefore, RTT is an example of how epigenetic effects in a person can vary over body regions and time. As such, *MeCP2* has been aptly referred to as a "moving target" for researchers based on the differences in expression and activity of MeCP2 depending on cell type and developmental time point (Feldman et al. 2016).

Possible treatment avenues for RTT have considered the neural mechanisms of the disorder to be potentially reversible. RTT is a syndrome of diminished MeCP2, but overexpression of *MeCP2* can also lead to neurological deficits (Lyst and Bird 2015). Therefore, MeCP2 levels require tight control. While studies continue to look for ways to directly treat MeCP2 dysfunction—through activating a silenced *MeCP2* (Przanowski et al. 2018), protein replacement, or various forms of gene therapy—treatment for RTT remains mostly geared toward symptom management, targeting the downstream effects of MeCP2 dysfunction.

15q11-q13 Deletion and Duplication Syndromes

Angelman syndrome and **Prader-Willi syndrome (PWS)**, two neurodevelopmental disorders often lumped together, have distinct patterns of symptoms. Individuals with Angelman syndrome are described as "happy puppets," with a persistently joyful demeanor accompanied by uplifted hand-flapping and facial dysmorphology; those affected by PWS do not carry these features (see Table 3–2). PWS is instead noted for marked hyperphagia with prominent obesity and atypical stature, among other symptoms. What makes these disorders remarkable, and the reason they are frequently discussed together, is their shared genetic and epigenetic etiology. Despite the striking differences in presentation, both disorders emerge from the blocked expression of precisely the same region of the chromosome. Parent-of-origin imprinting and subsequent loss of expression of otherwise functional genes lead to two clinically distinct disorders.

PWS has an estimated prevalence of one in 10,000–30,000 people and spans multiple body systems in affected individuals, with many symptoms linked to endocrine and hypothalamic dysfunction. During the neonatal period, the syndrome is consistently associated with severe hypotonia, lethargy, and difficulty with feeding. Those affected also exhibit

Table 3–2. Clinical insights: assessment and intervention in PWS and Angelman syndrome

Food-related issues in PWS

◆ Address food-related behaviors early. Behavioral problems and emotional dysregulation in PWS may arise from food preoccupations and lack of satiety. Interventions may include tight control of access to food, promoting a healthy/balanced diet, and encouraging routine exercise.

◆ It is undeniably crucial to start working with a dietitian early.

◆ Work with primary care or endocrinology to consider the use of exogenous growth hormone. It has been shown that strict, healthy diet plans help with normalizing body mass index; however, growth and height may be significantly impeded, and growth hormone may help.

Self-injurious behavior and aggression in 15q11-q13 deletion

◆ Aggression generally serves a purpose and is usually more pronounced in individuals with Angelman syndrome than those with PWS. This relationship correlates with a greater degree of cognitive impairment in Angelman syndrome.

◆ Behavioral problems may be triggered by

  ❖ Underlying medical concerns (e.g., headache, difficulty breathing, or pain);

  ❖ Hunger; or

  ❖ Difficulty in communicating other social needs.

◆ Interventions may include identifying the reason and intervening appropriately:

  ❖ Address the disturbance (for example, provide support or treatment for headache or other pain).

  ❖ Implement and teach other ways to communicate needs to adult caregivers, such as through the use of augmentative and alternative communication.

Communication concerns in 15q11-q13 deletion

◆ Communication impairment is greater in Angelman syndrome than in PWS: ~85% of individuals with Angelman syndrome exhibit significant deficits in speech production.

◆ Individuals with Angelman syndrome prefer nonverbal forms of communication (e.g., signing, facial expression, touching, eye contact, body movement, and posturing).

◆ The use of augmentative and alternative communication may be necessary to aid nonverbal communication.

Table 3–2.   Clinical insights: assessment and intervention in PWS
              and Angelman syndrome *(continued)*

    ❖ Evidence-Based Instructional Practices, hosted by Vanderbilt (Chazin et al. 2016), provides useful information on augmentative and alternative communication.

    ❖ Examples of augmentative and alternative communication include speech-generating devices, electronic tablet speech applications, homemade binders or books of picture symbols, and a picture exchange communication system.

◆ Speech-language pathology intervention should be performed early.

Seizures in Angelman syndrome

◆ Seizures are incredibly common: ~85% of those with Angelman syndrome experience them.

◆ Seizure types commonly seen in Angelman syndrome include generalized tonic-clonic, atypical absence, atonic, and myoclonic.

◆ Factors that may decrease seizure threshold include poor sleep or lack of sleep, an infectious process, dehydration, fever, emotional stress, or elevated sensory input.

Sleep disturbance in 15q11-q13 deletion

◆ Sleep disturbance can worsen daytime behavioral problems or increase risk of other concerns such as seizures. Some interventions to improve sleep pattern that may be recommended to patients and families:

    ❖ Keep a consistent sleep-wake schedule.

    ❖ Follow a relaxing bedtime routine, beginning about an hour before bedtime, with activities identified as soothing to the affected individual, such as calming music or a warm bath.

    ❖ Reduce the use of nonprescribed stimulants, including caffeine.

    ❖ Reduce daytime naps, especially in the afternoon, and keep the child engaged and active during the day.

    ❖ A sleep aid supplement or medication (e.g., melatonin, antihistamine, α-2 agonist) may be appropriate if other interventions fail.

Management of additional behavioral concerns in 15q11-q13 deletion

◆ A patient with Angelman syndrome or PWS may qualify for ABA therapy with an emphasis on differential positive reinforcement of other behavior.

◆ A practitioner may implement CBT techniques for skin picking and obsessive-compulsive behaviors, including habit reversal techniques and exposure and response prevention, if appropriate.

Table 3–2.　Clinical insights: assessment and intervention in PWS and Angelman syndrome *(continued)*

◆　SSRIs have been successful in this patient population, based on some small studies, for management of temper outburst and obsessive-compulsive symptoms.

◆　Judicious use of antipsychotics for management of behavioral issues may be considered, opting for those with the least likelihood of causing weight gain, as this is a major concern in PWS.

Note.　ABA=applied behavioral analysis; CBT=cognitive-behavioral therapy; PWS=Prader-Willi syndrome; SSRI=selective serotonin reuptake inhibitor.

thickened saliva, a disproportionately large head circumference with increased head/chest circumference ratio, and small genitalia. With age, global developmental delay becomes noticeable, as do short stature and decreased growth. In childhood, excessive eating (hyperphagia) leads to prominent obesity. In adolescence, there is exaggeration of typical teenager rebelliousness fueled by the need to obtain more food. Cognitive impairment remains alongside behavioral issues and obsessive-compulsive tendencies. Common concerns therefore include hyperphagia, nutrition, and obesity. Individuals with PWS may live well into adulthood but are susceptible to death by accidents, aspiration, choking, and sepsis in childhood and adolescence and cardiopulmonary, respiratory, and obesity-related morbidity in adulthood (Butler et al. 2017).

Like PWS, Angelman syndrome is rather uncommon, with an estimated prevalence of one in 12,000–20,000 (Williams et al. 2010). DSM-5-TR (American Psychiatric Association 2022) does not list diagnostic criteria for either PWS or Angelman syndrome, but criteria have been determined via consensus (Williams et al. 2006). Children with Angelman syndrome display certain patterns of face dysmorphology including microcephaly, deep-set eyes, pointed chin, wide mouth, protruding tongue, prognathia, and hypopigmented skin (Williams et al. 2006). Compared with the general population, children with Angelman syndrome demonstrate significant developmental delay, ongoing cognitive deficits, impaired speech, and autism-like behaviors. The developmental delay becomes apparent around 6–12 months of age and is preceded by unremarkable prenatal and birth history (Williams et al. 2010). Angelman syndrome is also commonly associated with seizures. Children with Angelman syndrome demonstrate an excitable affect, frequently smiling and laughing, and ataxia coupled with uplifted hand flapping. Because of these behavioral manifestations and appearance of the disorder, individuals affected by Angelman syndrome have been likened to "happy puppets." Those with Angelman syndrome have a relatively normal life span, but as they age, many continue to have seizures, sleep dysfunction, constipation, obesity, and self-injurious behavior (Larson et al. 2015).

Despite the differences in the phenotypes of PWS and Angelman syndrome, both are associated with silencing of genes located in a section of the long arm of chromosome 15, specifically 15q11-q13 (see Chapter 1, "Overview of Genetic and Epigenetic Mechanisms," for a review of relevant nomenclature and classification). This region is a hotspot for genes relevant for neurodevelopment, several of which are subject to genomic imprinting leading to parent-of-origin–specific expression (Depienne et al. 2009; Scoles 2011; Zink et al. 2018). As discussed in Chapter 1, imprinting occurs when the maternal and paternal chromosomes are marked before conception, with marks persisting through development, allowing the nuclear machinery to keep track of the parent-of-origin of each chromosome throughout the life span. As such, cells can select either the maternal or paternal chromosome for gene expression while silencing the other through epigenetic mechanisms under control of a nearby imprinting center (Lewis and Reik 2006). As such, in neural tissue, only one copy is expressed of some of the genes of 15q11-q13, while other tissues may express the genes from both parents. The selection of which copy to express is not random but is based on the parent-of-origin imprinting marks left on the chromosomes, where the imprinted gene is silenced. So, in that region, if the paternal copy is imprinted, then only the maternal copy can be expressed, and if the maternal copy is imprinted, only the paternal copy can be expressed.

Typical neurological development requires one functional copy of region 15q11-q13 from each parent. If an individual is missing one functional copy of this region from either parent—even if the other copy is completely unaffected—there is no compensatory action to express the imprinted genes from the other functional copy received. Therefore, if an individual receives a mutated gene within this chromosome segment from a parent, pathology arises if the wild-type (functional) gene is imprinted, as it cannot be expressed. Similarly, if an individual receives two copies of 15q11-q13 from one parent (as in the case of uniparental disomy), both sets of genes carry the same imprinting pattern, preventing the expression of those genes, while the nonimprinted genes are able to be expressed.

One gene that stands out as particularly important for the etiology of Angelman syndrome is *UBE3A*, which codes for a ubiquitin protein ligase involved in protein degradation pathways. Loss of function of this gene alone drives the development of Angelman syndrome in ~10% of cases, whereas a few other genes are involved in PWS.

Another disorder associated with this area, **15q11-q13 duplication syndrome (dup15q syndrome)**, occurs when individuals carry maternally and paternally imprinted copies of the chromosome and one copy contains a duplication of the genes in this region, leading to an increased copy number of the genes. Those affected by the syndrome show varying degrees of developmental delay with autism-like behaviors, motor impairment with hypotonia, language impairment, cognitive deficit, and seizures (Ajayi et al. 2017). Notably, it is the additional maternally expressed genes that lead to clinical presentations: paternal duplications are less likely to have notable neurodevelopmental sequelae (Copping et al. 2017). The pathology of dup15q syndrome provides a further example of how aberrant gene expression associated with this same region can lead to a distinct syndrome. Furthermore, it provides a hint about the importance of tight regulation of the expression of these genes in neural tissue, where both overexpression and underexpression lead to pathology.

PWS is understood to occur when the paternally expressed genes of 15q11-q13 have undergone mutation or are totally absent (a mnemonic is "p" for Prader-Willi and paternal absence). De novo mutation within this segment of the paternal chromosomal copy results in ~70% of cases of PWS. About 25% of cases of PWS result from an error in meiosis, where the offspring gets two copies of the maternal chromosome 15 with no paternal form, known as maternal uniparental disomy. Finally, ~1%–3% of cases of PWS result from an imprinting defect in the paternal copy.

Angelman syndrome (mnemonic: angel mom, maternal absence) follows a similar pattern of genomic defect in this region when instead the maternally expressed genes are dysfunctional or absent. Furthermore, as Angelman syndrome is tied primarily to *UBE3A*, mutations on that gene alone that spare the rest of 15q11-q13 can lead to the Angelman syndrome phenotype. About 10% of Angelman syndrome cases stem from a mutation of the maternally originating *UBE3A* gene, and ~70% occur as a result of a de novo deletion in 15q11-q13. Paternal uniparental disomy is a less common cause of Angelman syndrome, accounting for just 2%–5% of cases. The remaining 2%–4% of cases result from imprinting defects (Buiting 2010) or other unidentifiable molecular defects (Tan et al. 2011). The causes of the imprinting defects may be either a microdeletion or aberrant methylation patterns within the imprinting control center. Therefore, patients with imprinting defects may have received chromosomes with unaffected base sequences from each parent, but because of aberrant imprinting methylation patterns, genes are inappropriately silenced. Errors in the epigenetic methylation or imprinting patterns themselves are termed **epimutations**. See Figure 3–1 for a relative breakdown of the causes of PWS and Angelman syndrome.

The various causes discussed here of the genetic/epigenetic pathology underlying development of PWS and Angelman syndrome allow us to see not only how genetics and epigenetics work together, but also the line that separates the two. To this end, although PWS and Angelman syndrome are discussed as epigenetic disorders, it is important to note that most cases, as illustrated in Figure 3–1, are caused by errors in genetic processes. Uniparental disomy is caused by errors in meiosis. De novo deletions of large sections of chromosomes are caused by errors during chromosome crossovers and translocations. The remaining cases are due to imprinting defects, many initiated by aberrant methylation patterns, with only a small portion triggered by microdeletions within the imprinting control center.

There is currently no cure for PWS, Angelman syndrome, or dup15q. Some treatments are under evaluation, in addition to strategies for symptom management to improve outcomes and quality of life. Research directed at treating Angelman syndrome through enhancing expression of *UBE3A* or reversing imprinting effects has yet to provide promising treatment avenues (Bi et al. 2016). Therefore, current treatments are primarily supportive and require a multidisciplinary approach.

Fetal Alcohol Spectrum Disorder

Of disorders caused by in utero toxin exposures, **fetal alcohol syndrome (FAS)** is among the most recognizable. The effect of prenatal alcohol exposure is dose dependent, leading to a spectrum of developmental consequences encompassing physiological, neurocognitive, and behavioral outcomes, termed **fetal alcohol spectrum disorder (FASD)** (Lussier et al. 2017). FAS is on the most extreme end of FASD, following chronic, heavy alcohol use during gestation.

Currently, FASD is primarily diagnosed clinically, as no specific biomarker is available (see Table 3–3). FASD is characterized by neurodevelopmental delay, growth impairment, and facial dysmorphology (Chudley 2018). Primary or sentinel facial features of FASD include short palpebral fissure length, smooth philtrum, and thin upper lip (Chudley 2018). For a systematic process to assess sentinel facial features in FASD, see Astley and Clarren (2001). Additional features may include microcephaly, micrognathia, flattened nasal bridge, "railroad track" ears, and upturned nose. The neurodevelopmental deficits in FASD are broad and persist into adulthood. They include cognitive impairment, poor self-regulation,

A. Prader-Willi syndrome

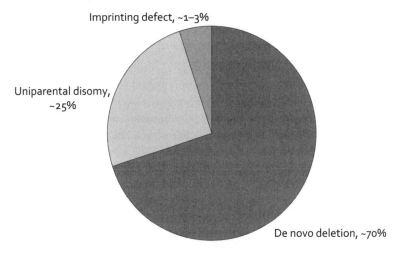

B. Angelman syndrome

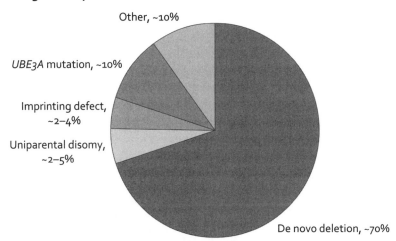

Figure 3–1. Genetic and epigenetic causes of Prader-Willi syndrome and Angelman syndrome.

Approximations of relative contributions of different genetic and epigenetic causes of Prader-Willi syndrome (**A**) and Angelman syndrome (**B**).

limited communication, and deficient activities of daily living (Lussier et al. 2017).

As with other specific neurodevelopmental disorders, DSM-5-TR (American Psychiatric Association 2022) does not define diagnostic criteria

Table 3–3. Clinical insights: assessment and intervention in fetal alcohol spectrum disorder

Assessment

◆ Although dysmorphic facial features are often considered a hallmark of FASD, an individual with the disorder may not exhibit any sentinel facial features. Therefore, definitive diagnosis may require a referral to a regional diagnostic specialist or team (which may include a behavioral pediatrician, geneticist, and neuropsychologist) that focuses on this disorder. There are also regional training centers for building expertise in this specific diagnosis.

◆ Encourage early assessment: early identification is associated with much better outcomes.

◆ Assess closely for signs of abuse or neglect, as this population is more prone to these traumatic events.

◆ Assess closely for treatable comorbid psychiatric conditions, such as depression, anxiety, or ADHD.

Treatment

◆ Anticipatory guidance

   ❖ Educate parents on the nature of cognitive deficits—including difficulties with executive function, impulsivity, working memory, spatial integration, and basic mathematics skills—to promote appropriate expectations.

   ❖ FASD is associated with increased risk in adolescence of criminal conduct and risky/sexual behaviors.

   ❖ Additional support is typically required in developing adaptive skills and activities of daily living.

   ❖ Early involvement in academic services (e.g., 504 plan [Section 504 of the Rehabilitation Act of 1973], IEP, special education) is recommended for improved outcomes.

◆ Build behavioral management techniques in the home through parent education, with an aim to increase stability and structure in the home, as well as incorporate simplified positive behavior rewards.

◆ Through case management, oversee family support including respite care, parent counseling, support groups, and resources for ongoing alcohol/drug abuse problems in the home.

◆ Promote development of social skills, including play dates at early ages and social skills programs, if available.

◆ Ensure proper assessment and monitoring for sequelae of FASD including cardiac defects, dental pathology, and deficiencies in vision, hearing, nutrition/growth, and sleep.

Table 3–3. Clinical insights: assessment and intervention in fetal alcohol spectrum disorder *(continued)*

◆ Investigate a possible role for OT, PT, SLP, and vocational training.

Additional resources

◆ The Fetal Alcohol Spectrum Disorders Program (American Academy of Pediatrics) includes an FASD toolkit, sample scripts, and other aids to implement clinically.

◆ CDC guidance on FASD includes regional training centers.

◆ FASD United provides information for families, support groups, and mentoring for mothers, as well as clinical resources for practitioners.

Note. FASD=fetal alcohol spectrum disorder; IEP=individualized education plan; OT=occupational therapy; PT=physical therapy; SLP=speech-language pathology.

for FASD but states that the specifier "associated with a known medical or genetic condition or environmental factor" be used when the individual's symptoms also meet criteria for ASD when FASD is determined. Also, if the individual's symptoms do not meet criteria for another diagnosis, "other specified neurodevelopmental disorder" may be used and specified as "neurodevelopmental disorder associated with prenatal alcohol exposure" (American Psychiatric Association 2022). Traditionally, diagnosis of FAS requires children to exhibit the three sentinel facial features with neurodevelopmental delay and impaired growth. Other discrete presentations within FASD may be found in the literature, such as partial fetal alcohol syndrome (pFAS), alcohol-related neurodevelopmental disorder (ARND), and neurobehavioral disorder associated with prenatal alcohol exposure (ND-PAE). More recent FASD diagnostic guidelines require known or possible alcohol exposure with subsequent central nervous system impairment (either assessed directly or presumed from the presence of microcephaly), with the classification options "FASD with sentinel facial features" or "FASD without sentinel facial features" (Cook et al. 2016).

Through different avenues of research, the mechanism has been determined by which prenatal alcohol exposure leads to the lifetime of effects: through changes in **fetal programming** (Lussier et al. 2017). Fetal programming refers to the effect that environment has in the developing fetus with respect to later pathology, through developmental, genetic, and epigenetic changes. *Fetal environment* most often refers to exposures in utero, including maternal hormone levels, nutritional availability, and toxin exposures. Prenatal alcohol exposure has been demonstrated to have epigenetic effects through changes in methylation, chromatin remodeling, and miRNAs (Lussier et al. 2017). Thus, the possible mechanism by which alcohol exposure during intrauterine development can lead to such significant and lasting changes is at least in part through modulating epigenetic function. Prenatal alcohol exposure has been shown to affect the availability of chromatin proteins, as well as histone modifications (Lussier et al. 2017).

In mouse models, high levels of prenatal alcohol exposure have been linked to globally decreased methylation over the genome (Garro et al. 1991). Notably, exposure to a DNA methylation inhibitor during embryogenesis leads to effects similar to those of alcohol exposure, with modulation of DNA methylation, and outcomes such as craniofacial deficits (Dasmahapatra and Khan 2015). Decreased DNA methyltransferase activity was proposed as a mechanism for the bulk change in DNA methylation, but as studies looked more closely at this effect, it became clear that this pattern of hypomethylation spanning the genome in FASD is only partially correct. Although a predominantly inhibitory trend toward gene expression affects genes of neurodevelopment in individuals with FASD, reduction in methylation is not uniform across tissues or even brain regions, as some brain regions and neural stem cells show increased methylation (Lussier et al. 2017; Zhou et al. 2011). Furthermore, in a study by Cobben et al. (2019) characterizing the genomewide DNA-methylation profile using peripheral blood samples from children with FASD versus children without in utero alcohol exposure, the findings revealed some areas with hypermethylation and others with hypomethylation. The authors focused on the 2,000 most differentially methylated positions and found a trend favoring hypermethylation across the genome of individuals affected by FASD (1,141 positions [~57%] hypermethylated; 859 [~43%] hypomethylated). The authors further noted that the positions of hypomethylation in FASD were more likely to be found in promoter regions and gene bodies, and positions of hypermethylation were more commonly found in the genes' first exons. Therefore, the epigenetic effects of alcohol exposure in utero may occur because of changes in the typical pattern of methylation across different tissues at different developmental time points. Further, the direction of methylation effect depends on timing of exposure, genes assessed, and even analysis method. In studies of human samples, both hypermethylation and hypomethylation have been found over multiple CpG sites, with undifferentiated cells more vulnerable to effects relative to differentiated cells, predominantly in promoter regions of chromosomes 2, 16, and 18 (Khalid et al. 2014; Laufer et al. 2015). Another study of methylation patterns showed that the majority of genes with altered methylation are highly expressed in the brain, and the genes themselves are understood to be involved in neurodevelopmental effects such as anxiety, epilepsy, and autism (Portales-Casamar et al. 2016). The authors also suggested that the pattern through which prenatal alcohol exposure alters typical methylation programs across the individual may be considered a biomarker for the disorder, an argument that was further strengthened in later studies (Lussier et al. 2018).

Noncoding RNA, miRNA, has also been studied as a mechanism through which alcohol leads to developmental effects. Notably, some of the miRNAs involved have been implicated in **neuroapoptosis**—the functional programmed death of neurons—suggesting the possible significance of this relationship. Exposure to alcohol showed effects (including upregulation and downregulation) on a variety of specific miRNAs (Lussier et al. 2017). Notably, in samples of peripheral blood from mothers with heavy alcohol use during pregnancy, 11 miRNAs were identified as elevated in affected infants compared with unaffected infants (Balaraman et al. 2016). In other words, whether alcohol exposure affects neurodevelopmental trajectories may be predicted by examining miRNA in maternal peripheral blood before the child is born. Another striking finding with respect to miRNA is that not only does alcohol exposure lead to effects, but alcohol withdrawal has its own unique effect on the epigenome, distinct from chronic exposure without withdrawal (Guo et al. 2012). Thus the dosing and timing of both alcohol exposure and its withdrawal may have lasting neurodevelopmental effects through epigenetic pathways.

In total, at the time of this writing, there is strong evidence for an epigenetic effect to explain the neurodevelopmental trajectory of FASD. The effect is complex, involving many different genes and different tissues in different ways, with no standout locus as yet. Regardless, it may be confidently asserted that global changes to methylation patterns and miRNA expression are strongly tied to the developmental pathway of the disorder. Additionally, possible treatment avenues for FASD are being informed by these epigenetic observations, including supplementation with choline to increase methyl availability, although findings have been mixed, and timing of administration may be essential (Nguyen et al. 2016; Thomas et al. 2007).

Trinucleotide Expansions: Fragile X Syndrome and Huntington's Disease

Fragile X Syndrome

Of the numerous syndromes characterized by intellectual disability, **fragile X syndrome (FXS)** stands out in part because its development has been tied to dysfunction of a single gene, known as **fragile X messenger ribonucleoprotein 1 (*FMR1*)**. Mutations of this gene are associated with a variety of phenotypic outcomes including autism, intellectual disability with delayed motor and language milestones, facial dysmorphology, tremor, ataxia, seizures, and primary ovarian insufficiency/premature ovarian failure (Hagerman et al. 2009). FXS is considered the most common known, heritable, single-gene disorder associated with autism spectrum disorder (ASD), and DSM-5-TR (American Psychiatric Association 2022) carries an additional specifier for ASD, "associated with a known medical or genetic condition or environmental factor," for which FXS may be indicated. FXS affects one in 3,600 males and one in 6,000 females (Hagerman et al. 2009). Although FXS is associated with some dysmorphic facial characteristics, those features may go unnoticed until the more prominent developmental delay and behavioral manifestations of the disorder become apparent. Physical features of FXS are understood to develop primarily from connective tissue dysplasia yielding a long and narrow face with high forehead, prominent jaw, and large ears. Additional findings include flat feet, hyperextensible joints, and macroorchidism in males.

FMR1 is located on the q (long) arm of the X chromosome and encodes **fragile X messenger ribonucleoprotein (FMRP)**. The mutation leading to these outcomes is a CGG trinucleotide repeat. The number of repeats is associated with emergence of symptoms: <45 CGG repeats is considered to be the normal variant, and >200 is a full mutation, typically associated with FXS. Expansions within this 45–200 range of repeats are termed **premutations**, with which individuals may show some symptomatology apart from FXS and carry a risk of transmitting a full mutation to their offspring. The premutation alleles, which are more common than full mutations, can become full mutations when maternally transmitted via expansion during meiosis. FMRP itself is an RNA-binding protein and therefore is understood to play a role in translational control and synthesis—and perhaps epigenetic regulation—of many proteins relevant for proper dendrite maturation, synaptic plasticity, and overall neurological development (Chen and Joseph 2015; Hagerman et al. 2009).

The full mutation, with >200 CGG repeats, is understood to create the phenotype of FXS through transcriptional silencing of *FMR1* (Pietrobono et al. 2002). However, some individuals with *FMR1* premutations demonstrate increased transcription of *FMR1*, with other syndromes arising later in life. One of them is fragile X–associated tremor/ataxia syndrome (FXTAS), which predominantly affects males and rarely females, emerges around age 50, and is characterized by tremors, gait instability, and falls. Males may also experience cognitive decline and dementia; females may demonstrate primary ovarian insufficiency/failure. Typically, individuals with the premutation demonstrate normal intelligence, although males may show cognitive dysfunction in attention, executive control, social deficits, and obsessive-compulsive behavior.

Although FXS is tied to a mutation in a single gene, the syndrome is relevant here because of the epigenetic effects that accompany the mutation. The location of the CGG repeat is upstream in the 5' untranslated region on *FMR1*, adjacent to the *FMR1* promoter region, which contains CpG islands. In FXS, both the CGG repeat and CpG island are hypermethylated, ultimately silencing *FMR1* at ~10–11 weeks' gestation (Mor-Shaked and Eiges 2018). The full mechanism may be more complex than transcriptional silencing by methylation alone (Colak et al. 2014). Research has shown, in addition, that in embryos, expression of *FMR1* may be impeded by RNA-DNA interaction. During transcription, if long enough (i.e., >200 CGG repeats), the transcribed RNA/mRNA may actually hook upstream, back toward the template DNA strand, and begin interacting with the still exposed Cs and Gs of the template DNA strand; such hybridization of the RNA-DNA is known as a **heteroduplex**. The formation of this complex leads to downstream transcriptional silencing pathways for *FMR1* (Colak et al. 2014).

More details on DNA methylation patterns in FXS have been documented. In addition to containing methylated CpG islands and CGG repeats, the *FMR1* promoter region has been shown to be flanked by epigenetic boundaries, named **fragile X–related elements 1 and 2 (FREE1 and FREE2)**, where FREE1 is upstream and FREE2 downstream of the promoter region. There is a notable transition from methylated DNA upstream of the boundary to unmethylated DNA downstream in non-affected individuals (Kraan et al. 2019). In FXS, methylation is found to cross these boundaries, transcending FREE1 and the entirety of the promoter region including the CpGs and transcription start site, CGG repeats, and FREE2. Increased methylation of these boundaries has been tied to decreased *FMR1* expression in the full mutation. Furthermore, some studies have shown a dose-dependent relationship of methylation in these regions, where higher levels of methylation of CpG islands and FREE2 were tied to degree of intellectual impairment and other symptom severity in individuals with FXS (Kraan et al. 2019).

In addition to decreased access of transcription factors to the over-methylated DNA, repressive histone modifications increase compaction of the chromatin, consequently reducing transcriptional activity. Further-more, studies have indicated a potential role of noncoding RNA (e.g., miRNA) in the silencing of *FMR1* in FXS (Zhou et al. 2019).

As with other disorders, these findings of epigenetic relationships within FXS have inspired pursuits to isolate treatment. Agents that re-move DNA methylation (5-azacytidine and 5-azadeoxycytidine) have par-tially reversed DNA methylation and histone modification at the *FMR1* locus in stem cells, although the effect did not last long after discontinu-ation of the otherwise cytogenic and mutagenic drugs (Kraan et al. 2019). Histone deacetylase (HDAC) inhibitors (notable examples being valproic acid and acetylcarnitine) have also been examined. Although these med-ications have not led to the same molecular effects as DNA demethylation agents (reactivating *FMR1*), trials have shown some improvement in hy-peractivity and other behaviors (but not intellectual functioning) with valproic acid and acetylcarnitine treatment. Therapeutic targets also in-clude reversing the epigenetic dysregulation at other sites resulting from loss of FMRP (Korb et al. 2017). Otherwise, treatment for FXS remains symptom focused and multidisciplinary, including speech therapy, phys-ical and occupational therapy, extensive school involvement with special education, and genetic counseling to support appropriate anticipation of an extensive family impact (Hagerman et al. 2009).

Huntington's Disease

Huntington's disease is a rare (5–10 cases per 100,000) but noteworthy neurodevelopmental disorder (see Table 3–4). Like other conditions de-scribed in this chapter, it is attributed to mutation of a single gene. Hun-tington's disease is characterized by gradual cognitive and motor decline with personality changes that occur later in life. The average age at symp-tom onset is 30–50 years, and the disease progresses over an average of 17–20 years before death (Roos 2010). Specifically, those with Huntington's disease begin to exhibit involuntary movements that begin in the distal extremities and ultimately progress to chorea, gait abnormality, and rigid-ity with contractures (Roos 2010). Psychiatric manifestations emerge be-fore motor symptoms, with the earliest sign being increased irritability, and later depression, suicidal ideation, anxiety, obsessive thoughts, compulsive behaviors, and eventually psychosis. Cognitive decline, most

Table 3–4. Clinical insights: assessment and intervention in Huntington's disease

Assessment

◆ Provide genetic counseling for the entire family, including predictive gene testing for offspring.

◆ Discuss advance directives early in anticipation of loss of capacity.

Treatment

◆ Treatment planning is primarily supportive, with symptom management through pharmacologic and nonpharmacologic means. Typical targets include chorea, dystonia, rigidity, pain, motor tics, dysphagia/aspiration, depression, agitation, and psychosis.

◆ A multidisciplinary team approach is needed to address neurologic symptoms (neurology), progression of physical impairments (physical therapy, occupational therapy, speech and language pathology), psychiatric symptoms, and impact on the family. Later stages of Huntington's disease may require home care services and palliative care.

◆ Discuss environmental modifications to increase the predictability and structure of the home, reduce stress, and limit physical obstacles to prevent falls.

Resources

◆ The Huntington's Disease Society of America includes multiple publications geared toward families and providers, with free electronic access.

◆ The International Huntington Association provides information for patients regarding Huntington's disease as well as direction toward resources across the globe.

notably in executive functioning, often begins before onset of motor symptoms, and leads to dementia with impaired memory but relatively spared language.

The **Huntingtin gene (*HTT*)**, located on chromosome 4, contains a repeating CAG segment within the coding region, specifically in exon 1. The CAG trinucleotide repeat may undergo expansion during gametogenesis, and as a result, offspring attain a greater number of CAG repeats in this gene than the parent-of-origin. The severity of symptoms and timing of onset have been shown to correlate with the number of CAG repeats, a phenomenon termed **anticipation**. Having 10–35 repeats is considered stable; an intermediate number of alleles (27–35 repeats) is described as unstable, with a risk of further lengthening during meiosis and transferring a diseased allele to offspring. Having 36–39 repeats may cause pathology, but not always; when it does, it is associated with later symptom emergence. At higher numbers of repeats (>40), disease onset comes at a younger age with nearly full penetrance. Transmission is autosomal dominant, so with just one *HTT* allele with >40 CAG repeats, the likelihood of expressing the phenotype is nearly 100%. Offspring inheriting the gene will express a more severe phenotype with earlier symptom onset. Juvenile onset may occur with >60 CAG repeats.

The mechanism by which *HTT* leads to pathology is also of note. The function of the HTT protein is complex, and CAG expansion is not understood to cause a loss of function; rather, the conformational structure of the protein seems to be what leads to pathology. The trinucleotide CAG is transcribed into the amino acid glutamine (Q); therefore, translated proteins have long chains of glutamine referred to as a polyglutamine (polyQ) region, which is considered neurotoxic. The reason for this toxicity is likely that the larger chain of glutamine affects the three-dimensional conformational structure of the protein; proteins with longer polyQ chains are more likely to interfere with cellular functions by aggregating to form inclusions in the nucleus, among other cellular compartments. Although the protein is expressed across a variety of tissues and brain regions, the pathology in Huntington's disease has primarily been attributed to effects on medium spiny neurons, which predominate the architecture of the caudate nucleus and putamen (Francelle et al. 2017). The caudate and putamen are components of the striatum within the basal ganglia. These regions of the brain are classically understood to be involved in reward processing, motor control, and cognition. Therefore, the motor, behavioral, and cognitive symptoms of Huntington's disease are largely explained by neurodegenerative effects in these brain regions. As the disease progresses, degeneration is seen more globally across the cortex.

Although individuals with a sufficient number of CAG repeats in *HTT* have a nearly 100% probability of developing Huntington's disease, pathology is not necessarily 100% explained by CAG repeats. A closer look shows that additional familial and environmental factors have a modulating effect. In the U.S.-Venezuela Collaborative Research Project—a massive study spanning nearly 25 years and including >18,000 individuals of Venezuelan families affected by Huntington's disease—researchers were able to statistically determine contributions of factors explaining the variance observed in age at onset of symptoms in Huntington's disease (Wexler et al. 2004). Although ~70% of the variance of age at onset was explained by number of CAG repeats, notable contributions from familial (or other genetic) factors and environmental factors explained the re-

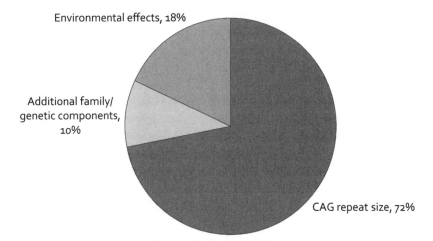

Environmental effects, 18%

Additional family/
genetic components,
10%

CAG repeat size, 72%

Figure 3–2. Factors affecting Huntington's disease age at onset.

Proportion of variance of contributing factors to the age at onset of Huntington's disease.

Source. Data from Wexler et al. (2004).

sidual proportion of variance. Shared and nonshared environmental effects contributed to a significant portion of this residual (see Figure 3-2). Therefore, despite the deterministic nature of having >40 CAG repeats in *HTT* with respect to developing Huntington's disease, there is more to be learned about the other genetic and environmental factors affecting the disorder. Considering these epigenetic changes in Huntington's disease related to pathology, it stands to reason that environmental factors may play a role in age at onset and disease progression. Such environmental factors have been found to be protective (increased physical activity and environmental enrichment) or harmful (substance abuse, stress, and sedentary lifestyle) (Thomas 2016). Furthermore, these environmental factors have been shown to drive epigenetic changes with downstream consequences on behavior, which may also be transmitted to the next generation.

Transcriptional dysregulation has been noted in Huntington's disease, with a research emphasis on a pattern of decreased histone acetylation (Francelle et al. 2017). Early findings demonstrated that the aggregates of HTT protein within the cell recruit transcription activators (specifically, the histone acetyltransferase cAMP response element-binding protein [CBP]) with subsequent change in pattern of the genes expressed in the neurons. The changes in gene expression follow a pattern that resembles that of more immature neurons. Additional research has shown that administration of HDAC inhibitors in animal models of Huntington's disease leads to increased histone acetylation in conjunction with decreased neuronal degeneration, improved motor function, and reduced lethality; however, this intervention is associated with significant side effects. See Francelle et al. (2017) for a more detailed review of the various ways histone modification has been demonstrated in Huntington's disease.

Enzymes that modulate histone methylation have also been shown to be dysregulated in Huntington's disease (Francelle et al. 2017). In particular, methylation of histone H3K9 is increased in the striatum and cortex, and methylation of histone H3K4 is decreased. Administration of nogalamycin, an antibiotic with chromatin-remodeling effects, reduces histone methylation (specifically H3K9me3), with subsequent decrease in heterochromatin condensation, and has been shown to slow Huntington's disease progression in mice (Lee et al. 2017). When neurons exhibited these epigenetic changes, the formation of nuclear inclusions characteristic of Huntington's disease was reduced, motor function was preserved, and life span was extended in the treated mice.

Through various study designs, DNA methylation patterns have also been demonstrated to be altered in Huntington's disease (Francelle et al. 2017). First of all, in neural tissue taken from mouse models, there is a global reduction in methylated cytosine (5-methylcytosine) and guanine (7-methylguanine). A closer look at the cells with the mutant *HTT* have shown changes to DNA methylation patterns specific to promoter regions of other genes that themselves have been shown to have altered expression in Huntington's disease. It has also been demonstrated that such DNA methylation changes may be tissue specific, linked to the higher degree of expression of *HTT* in the brain, and related to patient age at time of disease onset (De Souza et al. 2016). The authors suggested that this pattern of DNA methylation across tissue types may underlie the differential expression of *HTT* via an effect on the transcription factor CTCF.

Conclusion

The disorders discussed in this chapter provide a glimpse of different applications of epigenetics. We hope that the reader achieves not only a better understanding of the role that epigenetics can play in each disorder, but also a stronger familiarity with epigenetic processes in general. Understanding these examples may foster more effective consumption of research updates. Rett syndrome demonstrates the pathology that a global dysregulation of epigenetic processes can lead to. Angelman syndrome and PWS exemplify the process of genomic imprinting, whereby having a normal allele is not sufficient when that chromosome is silenced. FASD illustrates the various epigenetic paths that toxic environmental stimuli can take during early neurodevelopment. FXS and Huntington's disease exemplify how disorders tied to single genes are still strongly affected by epigenetic factors. A focus on the epigenetics of these disorders also provides a glimpse of potential future avenues of research that may inform more thorough understanding of pathogenesis and potential treatment options.

KEY POINTS

- Genetically, schizophrenia has been tied to variants at multiple gene sites, including common variants with low penetrance and uncommon variants with high penetrance. Epigenetically, a variety of DNA methylation patterns across the genome appear in people with schizophrenia. Although many epigenetic patterns differ widely between individuals with schizophrenia, some regions have emerged as relevant through single-gene and epigenomewide methylation studies, including *COMT*, *RELN*, and others relevant for metabolic/mitochondrial and inflammatory processes.

- Most cases of autism spectrum disorder (ASD) appear to arise from heritable and de novo genetic vulnerabilities interacting with environmental factors, where the majority of cases of ASD are not tied to a specific genetic abnormality. Higher folic acid intake before conception and through the first month of gestation has been linked to a lower incidence of ASD, possibly due to folate's role in DNA methylation. Epigenetic studies of ASD have found enrichment of CpG sites over identified ASD risk areas rather than DNA methylation changes consistent across ASD cases compared with unaffected controls.

- Rett syndrome (RTT) is caused by a single-gene mutation of methyl CpG-binding protein 2 (*MeCP2*), leading to a loss of function of the protein. Typically, MeCP2 binds to methylated cytosine of CpG islands of a variety of genes, such as *BDNF*, and so is essential to epigenetic regulation of gene expression. RTT is therefore a disorder caused by a gene mutation that leads to organism-wide dysfunction of epigenetic mechanisms.

- Angelman syndrome and Prader-Willi syndrome (PWS) are two neurodevelopmental disorders with quite different presentations despite both emerging from blocked expression of the same exact region of chromosome 15 (15q11-q13). The differences in symptoms and development result from parent-of-origin imprinting of genes: if the paternally expressed (maternally imprinted/silenced) gene of this region is absent or mutated, then PWS emerges. If the maternally expressed (paternally imprinted/silenced) gene of this region is absent or mutated, then Angelman syndrome emerges.

- Prenatal alcohol exposure has been demonstrated to have epigenetic effects through changes in methylation, chromatin remodeling, and miRNAs related to the developmental pathway of fetal alcohol spectrum disorder (FASD); the effect is complex, however. Both hypermethylation and hypomethylation have been found over multiple DNA CpG sites in response to in utero alcohol exposure. Some of the miRNAs affected by prenatal alcohol exposure are involved in neuroapoptosis, suggesting a possible mechanism, although both upregulation and downregulation of a variety of miRNAs have been found.

- Fragile X syndrome (FXS) is the most common inheritable single-gene disorder associated with autism spectrum disorder (ASD). FXS has been tied to dysfunction of a single gene, fragile X messenger ribonucleoprotein 1 (*FMR1*), in which a CGG trinucleotide repeat may expand and, through a variety of mechanisms, suppress an otherwise functional gene. The location of the CGG repeat is upstream from the coding region, providing additional potential methylation sites and allowing formation of an RNA-DNA heteroduplex during transcription, downregulating expression.

- Huntington's disease, a disorder tied to a trinucleotide repeat, is associated with a CAG variable-number repeat that occurs in the coding region of the Huntingtin gene (*HTT*). The repeat ends up being encoded in the protein as a series of glutamines, creating a polyQ region that affects the conformational structure of the protein, making it neurotoxic. The Huntington genotype has near-complete penetrance, meaning nearly 100% of individuals with the requisite number of CAG repeats in *HTT* go on to develop Huntington's disease; however, other familial and environmental factors affect development of pathology as well. Epigenetic effects through histone acetylation and methylation, as well as DNA methylation, have been found to affect regulation of *HTT* transcription.

Study Questions

1. Which gene located within 22q11 may have methylation differences tied to development of schizophenia?

    A. *UBE3A*
    B. *FMR1*
    C. *RELN*
    D. *COMT*

    Best answer: D

    Explanation: The catechol-*O*-methyltransferase (*COMT*) gene encodes an enzyme that breaks down catecholamines. Polymorphisms of *COMT* raise the risk of schizophrenia, and DNA methylation differences around *COMT* appear to impact expression in some individuals with the disorder. *COMT* is located within 22q11, further suggesting a role in velocardiofacial syndrome, with which a band within this section is deleted. *UBE3A* (answer A) is important to the development of Angelman syndrome and is found within the region of 15q11-15q13. *FMR1* (answer B) is tied to fragile X syndrome (and therefore located on the X chromosome, not chromosome 22). Disruption of DNA methylation of *RELN* (answer C) has been implicated in schizophrenia, but it is mapped to chromosome 7.

2. What process is deficient in Rett syndrome?

    A. Methyl-binding protein
    B. Imprinting
    C. Fetal programming
    D. DNA methyltransferase

    Best answer: A

    Explanation: The development of Rett syndrome is due to a loss of function of MeCP2, a methyl-binding protein involved heavily in the epigenetic regulation of several genes (answer A). Although the entire pathway from loss of MeCP2 to the phenotype of Rett syndrome is not fully known at this time, it is apparent that loss of this methyl-binding protein leads to problems in neurogenesis and neuronal migration and compromised synaptic plasticity, among other effects. Imprinting (answer B) is not known to play a role in

Rett syndrome but may be involved in PWS and Angelman syndrome. Dysfunction of fetal programming (answer C) refers more to environmental or in utero exposures in fetal development and applies to fetal alcohol spectrum disorder. DNA methyltransferases (answer D) are not understood to be a significant driving factor in the development of Rett syndrome.

3. Which of the following is the cause of Rett syndrome?

A. An inherited aberrant epigenetic methylation pattern
B. An error in X chromosome inactivation
C. A de novo gene mutation of *MeCP2*
D. Expansion of trinucleotide repeats of *MeCP2*

Best answer: C

Explanation: Rett syndrome is caused by a spontaneous, non-inherited (de novo) mutation of methyl CpG-binding protein 2 (*MeCP2*), a methyl-binding protein involved in epigenetic regulation of several other genes, as well as additional mechanisms (answer C). Therefore, although Rett syndrome is considered a neurodevelopmental disorder of epigenetic processes, it is actually caused by a single gene mutation. Rett syndrome is not inherited and is also caused by a problem with the epigenetic machinery's ability to use methylation patterns to regulate gene expression, rather than an issue with the epigenetic methylation pattern itself (answer A). X chromosome inactivation (answer B) does play a role in Rett syndrome, but it is not considered a cause, because the process functions properly (in the same way as in unaffected individuals). However, individuals with Rett syndrome typically have one functional and one dysfunctional copy of *MeCP2*, and because of random X chromosome inactivation, there is a 50/50 chance the cell will be able to produce a functional MeCP2 protein. There is no expansion of trinucleotide repeat (answer D) in Rett syndrome; that occurs in fragile X syndrome and Huntington's disease, among other disorders.

4. The majority of Prader-Willi syndrome (PWS) cases result from which of the following errors?

A. Imprinting error
B. Point mutation

C. Maternal uniparental disomy
D. Deletion within the region 15q11-q13

Best answer: D

Explanation: A majority (~70%) of cases of PWS and Angelman syndrome are caused by de novo deletions of chromosome region 15q11-q13 (answer D). Although imprinting plays a role in the development of PWS and Angelman syndrome, only a small portion of cases are caused by errors in imprinting (contradicting answer A). Most cases are caused by a deletion spanning a region of chromosome 15, and when the process of paternal imprinting functions properly, the genes that are inherited intact are not expressed. A point mutation (answer B) explains a proportion of Angelman syndrome cases, but not PWS cases: multiple genes within the region are implicated in PWS, but a majority of Angelman syndrome features arise from effects of a single gene. Uniparental disomy (answer C) is the second most common cause of PWS and explains a portion of Angelman syndrome cases. Uniparental disomy is associated with a nondisjunction error that occurs during meiosis wherein the offspring gets both copies of a chromosome from one parent, in this case chromosome 15 from the mother in PWS or from the father in Angelman syndrome. In imprinted genes, typically only one allele is expressed; the other is silenced (monoallelic expression). So, in cases of PWS due to maternal uniparental disomy, the maternal copies are silenced, and the paternal copy is absent owing to nondisjunction error.

5.　　A de novo mutation to which gene may lead to Angelman syndrome?

A. *MeCP2*
B. *UBE3A*
C. *Dup15q*
D. *HTT*

Best answer: B

Explanation: Angelman syndrome may be caused by a de novo mutation of the ubiquitin protein ligase E3A (*UBE3A*) gene (answer B). UBE3A is involved in protein degradation pathways and is located in the 15q11-q13 region. Although other maternally expressed genes are involved, *UBE3A* appears to contribute most substantially to the Angelman syndrome phenotype. Therefore, although no single gene mutation can cause PWS (but rather, a loss of function of multiple genes in the 15q11-q13 region is needed), it is possible for Angelman syndrome to emerge from a mutation of *UBE3A* alone, without affecting other genes in the 15q11-q13 region. Rett syndrome is caused by a de novo mutation of methyl CpG-binding protein 2 (*MeCP2*) (answer A). There is no "*dup15q* gene" (answer C); rather, dup15q is the shorthand name for duplication 15q11-q13 syndrome, with which an individual gains an extra copy of genes in this region from one parent (typically the mother), leading to overexpression, with subsequent developmental delay, autism-like features, and seizures. The Huntingtin gene, or *HTT* (answer D), includes a CAG repeat that may undergo expansion, leading to Huntington's disease.

6.   What percentage of cases of PWS and Angelman syndrome are caused by an error of epigenetic processes rather than an error of genetic processes?

A. <5%
B. 10%–15%
C. 25%–30%
D. >70%

Best answer: A

Explanation: Imprinting defects account for <5% of cases of PWS and Angelman syndrome (answer A). Furthermore, of those imprinting defects, a majority are caused by microdeletions at the imprinting center. This leaves only ~1% of total cases of both syndromes with unaffected gene sequences, to be explained entirely by inherited aberrant methylation patterns (epimutations). About 10% of Angelman syndrome cases (answer B) are explained by mutations to *UBE3A* alone. About 25% of PWS cases (answer C) are caused by maternal uniparental disomy. About 70% of cases of both PWS and Angelman syndrome (answer D) are attributed to deletions of the chromosome region 15q11-q13.

7.   With respect to development of fetal alcohol spectrum disorder (FASD), exposure to high levels of alcohol in utero is associated with

A. Global elevation in methylation across chromosomes
B. Global decrease in methylation across chromosomes
C. Global changes to methylation patterns, including increases in some chromosome locations and decreases in others
D. No change to methylation across chromosomes

Best answer: C

Explanation: In FASD, the expression of many genes of neurodevelopment appear to be affected, which occurs in part through decreased methylation in some portions of the chromosomes and increased methylation in others. There is a predominantly inhibitory trend toward gene expression skewed toward genes of neurodevelopment, but the epigenetic effects of alcohol exposure in utero are not simply of decreasing methylation on chromosomes, but rather through changing the typical pattern of methylation across the genome (answer C). Early studies of mouse models suggested globally decreased methylation over the genome (answer B)—not the best answer, because further research was able to better define this relationship as a pattern of increase in some regions and decrease in others. There have been no studies that suggest global increases in methylation (answer A) or no change in methylation (answer D) in individuals affected by FASD.

8.   What is the current understanding of how *FMR1* becomes inactivated?

A. The full mutation of the gene is silenced through X-inactivation at conception.
B. As the genome is transcribed, an RNA-DNA heteroduplex forms in the full mutation, leading to silencing pathways.
C. Fragile X–related elements 1 and 2 (FREE1 and FREE2) prevent methylation upstream from the *FMR1* promoter region of the full mutation.
D. The full mutation of *FMR1* is inactivated later in life (after age 50), leading to other syndromes such as fragile X–associated tremor/ataxia syndrome (FXTAS).

Best answer: B

Explanation: As transcription occurs, DNA is unwound and exposed. If *FMR1* is long enough (i.e., has >200 CGG repeats), then there is an increased chance that the mRNA transcript will hook back and interact with upstream portions of the DNA template strand. With the mRNA and DNA transcript in close proximity, as well as a relative abundance of cytosine and guanine bases that are apt to interact with each other spontaneously, the DNA template and mRNA transcript can form a rather stable complex known as an RNA-DNA heteroduplex. The formation of this heteroduplex is understood to lead to downstream silencing pathways for *FMR1* (answer B). In fragile X syndrome (FXS), the silencing of *FMR1* through heteroduplex takes some time, ~10–11 weeks of development in utero. Therefore, silencing occurs after conception and is not related to X-inactivation (answer A). FREE1 and FREE2 are epigenetic boundaries, where there is a notable transition from methylated DNA upstream of the boundary to unmethylated DNA downstream. In FXS with a full *FMR1* mutation, DNA upstream from FREE1 and FREE2 remains methylated; however, methylation is found to cross these boundaries, yielding higher levels of methylation downstream from their locations relative to unaffected individuals (answer C). The mechanism by which individuals develop FXTAS (answer D) is understood to require a premutation of *FMR1* (45–200 CGG repeats) and occurs by increased transcription of *FMR1*, as the symptoms arise later in life.

9. Which of the following is true regarding *FMR1* and FXS?

    A. *FMR1* includes a variable number of CAG repeats and is found on the X chromosome.
    B. The CGG repeats of *FMR1* are upstream from the coding region; therefore the number of repeats affects the expression of the gene, not the structure of the protein.
    C. Having <200 CGG repeats on *FMR1* is associated with a decreased risk of FXS but the same pathology when it occurs.
    D. *FMR1* contains fragile X–related elements 1 and 2 (FREE1 and FREE2), which act as epigenetic boundaries: individuals with FXS show no methylation crossing these boundaries.

Best answer: B

Explanation: In FXS, hypermethylation of both CpG islands and CGG repeats within the *FMR1* promoter region have been implicated in *FMR1* gene silencing. Both hypermethylation of these regions and the formation of RNA-DNA heteroduplex secondary to extended repeats in the promoter region contribute to a decrease in expression of the gene. The structure of the protein transcribed is unaffected by the number of CGG repeats (answer B). *FMR1* is located on the X chromosome and is considered sex linked. However, it includes a variable number of CGG repeats, not CAG repeats (answer A) as in the case of *HTT* and Huntington's disease. The premutation of *FMR1* (containing 45–200 CGG repeats) is associated with symptoms distinct from FXS (contradicting answer C), and individuals with this premutation carry a risk of transmitting the full mutation to their offspring. In FXS, methylation is found to cross the FREE1 and FREE2 boundaries flanking the *FMR1* promoter region (answer D), yielding higher levels of methylation downstream from their locations, into the CpG islands (FREE1) and into intron 1 (FREE2) of *FMR1*. Increased methylation of each of these sites with the *FMR1* CpG island are tied to decreased *FMR1* expression in the full mutation.

10.   Premutation of *FMR1* may lead to which of the following symptoms?

A. Tremors and ataxia in childhood in males
B. Cognitive decline beginning in adolescence
C. Microorchidism in males
D. Primary ovarian insufficiency in females

Best answer: D

Explanation: A premutation of *FMR1* refers to an expansion of CGG repeats, ~45–200. Premutations in *FMR1* may lead to pathology distinct from FXS. In males, this includes tremors, ataxia, and cognitive decline beginning later in adulthood, around age 50 (eliminating answers A and B). Females with *FMR1* premutations may demonstrate primary ovarian insufficiency and premature ovarian failure (answer D). Macroorchidism may occur in males with FXS; microorchidism (answer C) is associated with other genetic disorders, including PWS.

11.   Which of the following is true regarding *HTT* and Huntington's disease?

A. *HTT* includes a variable number of CAG repeats and is found on the X chromosome.

B. The CAG repeats of *HTT* are upstream from the coding region, and therefore the number of repeats affects the expression of the gene, not the structure of the protein.

C. Although having a sufficient number of CAG repeats on *HTT* is associated with a nearly 100% chance of developing Huntington's disease, there are environmental effects that contribute to the age at symptom onset.

D. When controlling for CAG repeat size on *HTT*, no other familial or genetic components contribute to age at symptom onset.

Best answer: C

Explanation: Individuals with a sufficient number of CAG repeats in *HTT* have a nearly 100% probability of developing Huntington's disease, but pathology is not 100% explained by number of CAG repeats. Additional familial and environmental factors have a modulating effect on development of pathology (answer C). *HTT* does include a variable number of CAG repeats (answer A), but it is located on chromosome 4 and is not sex linked. CAG repeats are in the coding region of *HTT*, so the Huntingtin protein contains an elongated polyglutamine (polyQ) region, making the transcribed protein neurotoxic (contradicting answer B). CAG repeat size accounts for ~70% of variance in age at onset; 10% is attributed to additional familial genetic components; and ~20% is tied to environmental effects (eliminating answer D).

References

Abrahams BS, Arking DE, Campbell DB, et al: SFARI Gene 2.0: a community-driven knowledgebase for the autism spectrum disorders (ASDs). Mol Autism 4(1):36, 2013

Ajayi OJ, Smith EJ, Viangteeravat T, et al, Dup15q Alliance: Multisite semiautomated clinical data repository for duplication 15q syndrome: study protocol and early uses. JMIR Res Protoc 6(10):e194, 2017 29046268

American Psychiatric Association: Diagnostic and Statistical Manual of Mental Disorders, 5th Edition, Text Revision. Arlington, VA, American Psychiatric Association, 2022

Andrews SV, Sheppard B, Windham GC, et al: Case-control meta-analysis of blood DNA methylation and autism spectrum disorder. Mol Autism 9(1):40, 2018

Astley SJ, Clarren SK: Measuring the facial phenotype of individuals with prenatal alcohol exposure: correlations with brain dysfunction. Alcohol Alcohol 36(2):147–159, 2001 11259212

Avramopoulos D: Recent advances in the genetics of schizophrenia. Mol Neuropsychiatry 4:35–51, 2018

Bakulski KM, Dou JF, Feinberg JI, et al: Autism-associated DNA methylation at birth from multiple tissues is enriched for autism genes in the early autism risk longitudinal investigation. Front Mol Neurosci 14:775390, 2021

Balaraman S, Schafer JJ, Tseng AM, et al: Plasma miRNA profiles in pregnant women predict infant outcomes following prenatal alcohol exposure. PLoS One 11(11):e0165081, 2016 27828986

Bi X, Sun J, Ji AX, Baudry M: Potential therapeutic approaches for Angelman syndrome. Expert Opin Ther Targets 20(5):601–613, 2016 26558806

Buiting K: Prader-Willi syndrome and Angelman syndrome. Am J Med Genet C Semin Med Genet 154C(3):365–376, 2010 20803659

Butler MG, Manzardo AM, Heinemann J, et al: Causes of death in Prader-Willi syndrome: Prader-Willi Syndrome Association (USA) 40-year mortality survey. Genet Med 19(6):635–642, 2017 27854358

Chase KA, Gavin DP, Guidotti A, Sharma RP: Histone methylation at H3K9: evidence for a restrictive epigenome in schizophrenia. Schizophr Res 149(1–3):15–20, 2013

Chazin KT, Quinn ED, Ledford JR: Augmentative and alternative communication (AAC), in Evidence-Based Instructional Practices for Young Children With Autism and Other Disabilities. Institute of Education Scientists, 2016. Available at: http://ebip.vkcsites.org/augmentative-and-alternative-communication. Accessed September 22, 2023.

Chen CH, Cheng MC, Hu TM, Ping LY: Chromosomal microarray analysis as first-tier genetic test for schizophrenia. Front Genet 12:620496, 2021

Chen E, Joseph S: Fragile X mental retardation protein: a paradigm for translational control by RNA-binding proteins. Biochimie 114:147–154, 2015 25701550

Chong HY, Teoh SL, Wu DBC, et al: Global economic burden of schizophrenia: a systematic review. Neuropsychiatr Dis Treat 12:357–373, 2016

Chudley AE: Diagnosis of fetal alcohol spectrum disorder: current practices and future considerations. Biochem Cell Biol 96(2):231–236, 2018 28746809

Ciernia AV, LaSalle J: The landscape of DNA methylation amid a perfect storm of autism aetiologies. Nat Rev Neurosci 17(7):411–423, 2016

Cobben JM, Krzyzewska IM, Venema A, et al: DNA methylation abundantly associates with fetal alcohol spectrum disorder and its subphenotypes. Epigenomics 11(7):767–785, 2019 30873861

Colak D, Zaninovic N, Cohen MS, et al: Promoter-bound trinucleotide repeat mRNA drives epigenetic silencing in fragile X syndrome. Science 343(6174):1002–1005, 2014 24578575

Cook JL, Green CR, Lilley CM, et al: Fetal alcohol spectrum disorder: a guideline for diagnosis across the lifespan. CMAJ 188(3):191–197, 2016 26668194

Copping NA, Christian SGB, Ritter DJ, et al: Neuronal overexpression of Ube3a isoform 2 causes behavioral impairments and neuroanatomical pathology relevant to 15q11.2-q13.3 duplication syndrome. Hum Mol Genet 26(20):3995–4010, 2017 29016856

Dasmahapatra AK, Khan IA: DNA methyltransferase expressions in Japanese rice fish (Oryzias latipes) embryogenesis is developmentally regulated and modulated by ethanol and 5-azacytidine. Comp Biochem Physiol C Toxicol Pharmacol 176–177:1–9, 2015 26183885

Depienne C, Moreno-De-Luca D, Heron D, et al: Screening for genomic rearrangements and methylation abnormalities of the 15q11-q13 region in autism spectrum disorders. Biol Psychiatry 66(4):349–359, 2009 19278672

De Souza RA, Islam SA, McEwen LM, et al: DNA methylation profiling in human Huntington's disease brain. Hum Mol Genet 25(10):2013–2030, 2016 26953320

Feldman D, Banerjee A, Sur M: Developmental dynamics of Rett syndrome. Neural Plast 2016:6154080, 2016 26942018

Francelle L, Lotz C, Outeiro T, et al: Contribution of neuroepigenetics to Huntington's disease. Front Hum Neurosci 11:17, 2017 28194101

Fusar-Poli P, Tantardini M, De Simone S, et al: Deconstructing vulnerability for psychosis: meta-analysis of environmental risk factors for psychosis in subjects at ultra high-risk. Eur Psychiatry 40:65–75, 2017

Garro AJ, McBeth DL, Lima V, Lieber CS: Ethanol consumption inhibits fetal DNA methylation in mice: implications for the fetal alcohol syndrome. Alcohol Clin Exp Res 15(3):395–398, 1991 1877725

Guo Y, Chen Y, Carreon S, Qiang M: Chronic intermittent ethanol exposure and its removal induce a different miRNA expression pattern in primary cortical neuronal cultures. Alcohol Clin Exp Res 36(6):1058–1066, 2012 22141737

Hagerman RJ, Berry-Kravis E, Kaufmann WE, et al: Advances in the treatment of fragile X syndrome. Pediatrics 123(1):378–390, 2009 19117905

Hilker R, Helenius D, Fagerlund B, et al: Heritability of schizophrenia and schizophrenia spectrum based on the nationwide Danish Twin Register. Biol Psychiatry 83(6):492–498, 2018

Horvath PM, Monteggia LM: MeCP2 as an activator of gene expression. Trends Neurosci 41(2):72–74, 2018 29405930

Khalid O, Kim JJ, Kim HS, et al: Gene expression signatures affected by alcohol-induced DNA methylomic deregulation in human embryonic stem cells. Stem Cell Res (Amst) 12(3):791–806, 2014 24751885

Korb E, Herre M, Zucker-Scharff I, et al: Excess translation of epigenetic regulators contributes to fragile X syndrome and is alleviated by Brd4 inhibition. Cell 170(6):1209–1223.e20, 2017 28823556

Kraan CM, Godler DE, Amor DJ: Epigenetics of fragile X syndrome and fragile X-related disorders. Dev Med Child Neurol 61(2):121–127, 2019 30084485

Larson AM, Shinnick JE, Shaaya EA, et al: Angelman syndrome in adulthood. Am J Med Genet A 167A(2):331–344, 2015 25428759

Laufer BI, Kapalanga J, Castellani CA, et al: Associative DNA methylation changes in children with prenatal alcohol exposure. Epigenomics 7(8):1259–1274, 2015 26178076

Lee J, Hwang YJ, Kim Y, et al: Remodeling of heterochromatin structure slows neuropathological progression and prolongs survival in an animal model of Huntington's disease. Acta Neuropathol 134(5):729–748, 2017 28593442

Lewis A, Reik W: How imprinting centres work. Cytogenet Genome Res 113(1–4):81–89, 2006 16575166

Lisoway AJ, Chen CC, Zai CC, et al: Toward personalized medicine in schizophrenia: genetics and epigenetics of antipsychotic treatment. Schizophr Res 232:112–124, 2021

Lussier AA, Weinberg J, Kobor MS: Epigenetics studies of fetal alcohol spectrum disorder: where are we now? Epigenomics 9(3):291–311, 2017 28234026

Lussier AA, Morin AM, MacIsaac JL, et al: DNA methylation as a predictor of fetal alcohol spectrum disorder. Clin Epigenetics 10:5, 2018 29344313

Lyst MJ, Bird A: Rett syndrome: a complex disorder with simple roots. Nat Rev Genet 16(5):261–275, 2015 25732612

Marconi A, Di Forti M, Lewis CM, et al: Meta-analysis of the association between the level of cannabis use and risk of psychosis. Schizophr Bull 42(5):1262–1269, 2016

Marshall CR, Howrigan DP, Merico D, et al: Contribution of copy number variants to schizophrenia from a genome-wide study of 41,321 subjects. Nat Genet 49(1):27–35, 2017

Mordaunt CE, Jianu JM, Laufer BI, et al: Cord blood DNA methylome in newborns later diagnosed with autism spectrum disorder reflects early dysregulation of neurodevelopmental and X-linked genes. Genome Med 12(1):88, 2020

Mor-Shaked H, Eiges R: Reevaluation of FMR1 hypermethylation timing in fragile X syndrome. Front Mol Neurosci 11:31, 2018 29467618

Nguyen TT, Risbud RD, Mattson SN, et al: Randomized, double-blind, placebo-controlled clinical trial of choline supplementation in school-aged children with fetal alcohol spectrum disorders. Am J Clin Nutr 104(6):1683–1692, 2016 27806977

Pietrobono R, Pomponi MG, Tabolacci E, et al: Quantitative analysis of DNA demethylation and transcriptional reactivation of the FMR1 gene in fragile X cells treated with 5-azadeoxycytidine. Nucleic Acids Res 30(14):3278–3285, 2002 12136110

Portales-Casamar E, Lussier AA, Jones MJ, et al: DNA methylation signature of human fetal alcohol spectrum disorder. Epigenetics Chromatin 9:25, 2016 27358653

Przanowski P, Wasko U, Zheng Z, et al: Pharmacological reactivation of inactive X-linked Mecp2 in cerebral cortical neurons of living mice. Proc Natl Acad Sci USA 115(31):7991–7996, 2018 30012595

Psychiatric Genomics Consortium: Meta-analysis of GWAS of over 16,000 individuals with autism spectrum disorder highlights a novel locus at 10q24.32 and a significant overlap with schizophrenia. Autism Spectrum Disorders Working Group. Mol Autism 8:21, 2017

Qiu Z: Deciphering MECP2-associated disorders: disrupted circuits and the hope for repair. Curr Opin Neurobiol 48:30–36, 2018 28961504

Richetto J, Meyer U: Epigenetic modifications in schizophrenia and related disorders: molecular scars of environmental exposures and source of phenotypic variability. Biol Psychiatry 89(3):215–226, 2021

Ripke S, Neale BM, Corvin A, et al: Biological insights from 108 schizophrenia-associated genetic loci. Nature 511(7510):421–427, 2014

Roos RA: Huntington's disease: a clinical review. Orphanet J Rare Dis 5:40, 2010 21171977

Roth TL, Lubin FD, Funk AJ, and Sweatt JD: Lasting epigenetic influence of early-life adversity on the BDNF gene. Biol Psychiatry 65(9):760–769, 2009

Scoles HA: Genetic and Epigenetic Alterations Within Chromosome 15q11–13.3 Affect Gene Expression in Human Neurodevelopmental Disorders. Master's thesis, University of California, Davis, 2011

Section 504 of the Rehabilitation Act of 1973: Handicapped Persons Rights Under Federal Law. Washington, DC: Department of Health, Education, and Welfare, Office of the Secretary, Office for Civil Rights, 1973

Sharma RP, Feiner B, Chase KA: Histone H3 phosphorylation is upregulated in PBMCs of schizophrenia patients in comparison to healthy controls. Schizophr Res 169(1–3):498–499, 2015

Singh T, Kurki MI, Curtis D, et al: Rare loss-of-function variants in SETD1A are associated with schizophrenia and developmental disorders. Nat Neurosci 19(4):571–577, 2016

Siu MT, Butcher DT, Turinsky AL, et al: Functional DNA methylation signatures for autism spectrum disorder genomic risk loci: 16p11.2 deletions and CHD8 variants. Clin Epigenet 11(1):103, 2019

Smigielski L, Jagannath V, Rössler W, et al: Epigenetic mechanisms in schizophrenia and other psychotic disorders: a systematic review of empirical human findings. Mol Psychiatry 25(8):1718–1748, 2020

Tan WH, Bacino CA, Skinner SA, et al: Angelman syndrome: mutations influence features in early childhood. Am J Med Genet A 155A(1):81–90, 2011 21204213

Thomas EA: DNA methylation in Huntington's disease: implications for transgenerational effects. Neurosci Lett 625:34–39, 2016 26522374

Thomas JD, Biane JS, O'Bryan KA, et al: Choline supplementation following third-trimester-equivalent alcohol exposure attenuates behavioral alterations in rats. Behav Neurosci 121(1):120–130, 2007 17324056

Torrey EF, Torrey BB, Peterson MR: Seasonality of schizophrenic births in the United States. Arch Gen Psychiatry 34(9):1065–1070, 1977

Villard L, Kpebe A, Cardoso C, et al: Two affected boys in a Rett syndrome family: clinical and molecular findings. Neurology 55(8):1188–1193, 2000 11071498

Wexler NS, Lorimer J, Porter J, et al: Venezuelan kindreds reveal that genetic and environmental factors modulate Huntington's disease age of onset. Proc Natl Acad Sci USA 101(10):3498–3503, 2004

Williams CA, Beaudet AL, Clayton-Smith J, et al: Angelman syndrome 2005: updated consensus for diagnostic criteria. Am J Med Genet A 140(5):413–418, 2006 16470747

Williams CA, Driscoll DJ, Dagli AI: Clinical and genetic aspects of Angelman syndrome. Genet Med 12(7):385–395, 2010 20445456

Woodward ND, Heckers S: Brain structure in neuropsychologically defined subgroups of schizophrenia and psychotic bipolar disorder. Schizophr Bull 41(6):1349–1359, 2015

Yang AC, Tsai SJ: New targets for schizophrenia treatment beyond the dopamine hypothesis. Int J Mol Sci, 2017

Zhou FC, Zhao Q, Liu Y, et al: Alteration of gene expression by alcohol exposure at early neurulation. BMC Genomics 12:124, 2011 21338521

Zhou Y, Hu Y, Sun Q, Xie N: Non-coding RNA in fragile X syndrome and converging mechanisms shared by related disorders. Front Genet 10:139, 2019 30881383

Zink F, Magnusdottir DN, Magnusson OT, et al: Insights into imprinting from parent-of-origin phased methylomes and transcriptomes. Nat Genet 50(11):1542–1552, 2018 30349119

Epigenetics of Childhood Trauma and Resilience

Kyle J. Rutledge, D.O., Ph.D.
Kai Anderson, M.D.
Onoriode Edeh, M.D.

The field of developmental neurobiology has long been dedicated to delineating the relationship between the environment and the brain. In brief, according to a well-established concept, neural networks follow a genetically programmed blueprint of development that is honed in an experience-dependent maturation process. This process of environmentally driven tuning of neural networks, with subsequent impact on behavior, is often referred to as **adaptation** (or **maladaptation** in the case of toxic environmental experiences) and has been found to incorporate epigenetic mechanisms.

In the field of psychiatry, we see over and over that illness and mental illness can be a consequence of traumatic experiences in early life. This understanding has steadily grown since the seminal Adverse Childhood Experiences (ACEs) studies of the late 1990s (Felitti et al. 1998). Since then, studies have shown that childhood adversity robustly contributes to development of mood, anxiety, behavior, and substance use disorders, emerging at any point across childhood, adolescence, or adulthood (Green et al. 2010). Furthermore, effects of early adverse experiences may later manifest as PTSD, eating disorders, or personality effects, with possible development of borderline or antisocial personality traits. Individuals with trauma history often face a variety of chronic medical illnesses as well as earlier mortality. In this chapter, we review pertinent physiology related to the body's stress response and potential downstream consequences on mental health. The overview includes a focus on glucocorticoid receptors and key regulation proteins, which have provided the most robust evidence for a potential role of epigenetics in environmentally driven neurobiological development. Next is an in-depth look at various presentations of stress and the correlations with epigenetic changes. We focus on early childhood trauma as well as preconception trauma, with a focus on **resilience** in stress responses.

Stress and Trauma

The term **stress** is rather broad, generally referring to some force or event that disrupts one's homeostasis. When understanding the effects of stress, two key elements must be considered: the stressor and the stress response. Stressors come in many forms, varying in intensity and duration, and may also include threats of harm or deprivation of needs. Stress responses include physiological actions occurring in tandem with protective behaviors (fighting, fleeing, freezing, associating, submitting, etc.) necessary to maintain homeostasis. Coping well with stress, then, is exhibiting an appropriate stress response for the right amount of time.

Early exposure to prolonged, frequent, or intense adversity, sometimes referred to as **toxic stress**, can have profound effects on a person's development. In psychiatry, we often refer to high-intensity stressors as **trauma** and speak in terms of acute or chronic durations of exposure. The pathway from toxic stress or trauma to its outcomes is multifactorial. Stress may impact people directly, by the physiological response of the trauma itself, and indirectly, by consequences of the adverse events, such as disrupted attachment styles, learned behavioral dynamics (which are adaptive in the stressed environment but maladaptive elsewhere), instability in the home or outlying environment, gravitation toward substance misuse, and extralegal involvement.

It is important to note that not all stress is bad. The classic Yerkes-Dodson law indicates that performance on an activity is going to be poor in situations of both too-high and too-low arousal (or stress), such that there is an optimal level of stimulation required to yield the best results (Broadhurst 1957). Similarly, during child development, cognitive and physical challenges drive positive development as the infant seeks more stimulating aspects of the environment, requiring more physical strength, better coordination, more efficient social communication, and more adept cognitive strategies to navigate. This idea of moderation being key may hold true for adversity, too. It is perhaps instinctive for people to shield themselves and their children from significant stressors, but the notion of *stress inoculation* not only has found a place in early developmental research but also has formed the foundation for some styles of psychotherapy designed for trauma disorders. The idea is that small, manageable stressors in the here and now can improve adaptive functioning—and, in turn, resilience—to better handle large, challenging stressors later. In the developmental literature, research involving rodents and humans consistently shows how early exposure to moderately distressing stimuli may lead to decreases in later anxiety responses with respect to both behavioral and physiological responses to stress. Regardless, the focus of this chapter is the too-high variety of stress.

A framework often incorporated into discussions of the development of stress-related pathology is the **diathesis-stress model** of disease development, which highlights the interactive effect of one's underlying predisposition to disease (diathesis) with the degree of exposure to stress. Individuals with a high predisposition to disease development may require only low levels of environmental stress to manifest a disorder, whereas high enough levels of stress can elicit pathology whether a person carries a low or high predisposition to disease. Applying this concept to stress, a dysfunctional stress response system may be considered a high predisposition to developing disease, including mental illness. But no matter how functional the stress response is, excessive activation will begin to cause deleterious consequences. In other words, having an overactive or underactive stress response can have a negative impact, as can a normal stress response that is activated to an extreme degree.

The diathesis-stress model of disease may be considered a specific application of "nature versus nurture" or gene and environment (GxE) interaction. As such, response to trauma stemming from the environment is strongly related to biological preparedness, informed by genetics. As this framework is informative but not exhaustive, later models began including coping strategies as an additional buffer to the interaction (GxExC). Recently, the role of epigenetics has been added as well; the most up-to-date representation of the model is (epi)GxExC (Schiele and Domschke 2018). Individuals exposed to toxic stress may exhibit changes in brain circuitry that can lead to dysfunction in emotion regulation, cognition, and behaviors, with subsequently increased risk of developing physical and mental illness. Research into the effects of environmental stress has uncovered the presence of complex epigenetic mechanisms that may play a role in these effects on human physiology and disease development.

Physiology of Stress

The **hypothalamic-pituitary-adrenal axis (HPA axis)** forms the core of the physiological stress response. The HPA axis, which includes the hypothalamus, pituitary gland, and adrenal glands, is a hormone-secreting neuroendocrine chain that tightly feeds back on itself. Both the hypothalamus and the pituitary gland are located above the brain stem; the adrenal glands rest above each kidney. The function of the HPA axis is regulated centrally through other brain regions, as well as parasympathetic and sympathetic systems. The body's initial reaction to stress is the acute release of epinephrine and norepinephrine, which helps prepare organs for distress. This event is followed by activation of the HPA axis. Beginning with the experience of a stressful event, the paraventricular nucleus of the hypothalamus releases two neuropeptides: corticotropin-releasing hormone (CRH) and arginine vasopressin (AVP). Both CRH and AVP then stimulate the release of adrenocorticotropic hormone (ACTH) from the anterior pituitary. ACTH stimulates the adrenal cortex with subsequent releases of glucocorticoid hormones including cortisol. Cortisol activates glucocorticoid receptors throughout the body (see Table 4–1), driving the body's stress response through a variety of mechanisms such as increased glucose availability to meet cell needs during stress states. In a negative feedback mechanism, release of high levels of cortisol into the bloodstream subsequently dials down HPA activity by binding to glucocorticoid receptors of the hypothalamus and anterior pituitary.

Although the neurophysiology of the stress response depends on the HPA axis, additional brain regions play key roles through their connections with the paraventricular nucleus of the hypothalamus (see Jankord and Herman [2008] and Nicolaides et al. [2015] for in-depth reviews). Notable regions include those that comprise the corticolimbic system: the prefrontal cortex, the amygdala, and the hippocampus. Through complex interactions, as well as interconnections of these areas with other regions of the brain, the experience of stress becomes highly complicated. Stress activation in the body may stem from a psychogenic stimulus rather than one from the external environment. And in stressful environmental situations, activity of the HPA axis may even be adaptively suppressed, contributing to resilience (Averill et al. 2018; Feder et al. 2009). Depending on the functioning at each of these neuroanatomical levels, we see different levels of activation or suppression of the HPA axis with stress. As a

Table 4–1.   Overview of glucocorticoid receptors

The glucocorticoid receptor is found across a wide variety of cells throughout the body, including neurons of the corticolimbic system comprising the prefrontal cortex, amygdala, and hippocampus. Glucocorticoid receptors may be referred to in the literature as NR3C1, from the nomenclature classifying steroid receptors (nuclear receptor, subfamily 3, group C, member 1). There are several endogenous glucocorticoids, although the predominant form in humans is cortisol (hydrocortisone). Glucocorticoid receptors are involved in metabolism, cell division, and a variety of other cellular functions, but here we focus on its role in the stress response.

Glucocorticoids are hydrophobic, so they may pass freely across the cell membrane to interact with their receptor in the cytoplasm. As with other steroid receptors in the body, glucocorticoid receptors are intracellular. Glucocorticoid receptors form stable complexes with heat shock proteins within the cytosol. Once binding to a glucocorticoid occurs, the dynamics of the complex become altered, enhancing both dissociation from the heat shock protein and translocation of the activated ligand-receptor complex into the nucleus, where it may influence transcription (Nicolaides et al. 2015). Outside the nucleus, the activated receptor may block potential transcription factors from entering the nucleus, thus regulating targeted gene expression. Inside the nucleus, the activated glucocorticoid receptor can bind to a section of the DNA known as the glucocorticoid response element (GRE). GREs are located in the promoter regions of a variety of genes. Whether transcription of the gene is increased or decreased after binding depends on other ligands bound to the activated glucocorticoid receptor.

FK506 binding protein 51 (FKBP5) modulates the stress response through its interaction with the glucocorticoid receptor. The relationship between FKBP5 and the glucocorticoid receptor is complex (see Zannas et al. [2016] for a review), but in short, FKBP5 plays a generally inhibitory role on glucocorticoid effects. FKBP5 may bind to the glucocorticoid receptor complex, delaying translocation into the nucleus, decreasing affinity for the glucocorticoid, and thus attenuating effects of the hormone. FKBP5 further inhibits glucocorticoid activity indirectly, through interactions with several other signaling pathways (Zannas et al. 2016). Notably, the promoter region of *FKBP5* itself has its own GRE, so its transcription can be induced by the presence of activated glucocorticoid receptors. Beyond interaction with the glucocorticoid receptor, FKBP5 has the potential to interact with several other major proteins, including calcineurin (a protein phosphatase that regulates synaptic transmission) and nuclear factor-κB (a transcription factor relevant for immune response and inflammation pathways).

result, different stressors in the same person may yield different effects, just as the same stressors in different people may yield different effects.

The negative feedback system that shuts down the stress response is critical for achieving homeostasis, and the activity of glucocorticoid receptors is integral to that system. When the strength of the inherent feedback mechanism is reduced, levels of stress hormones become pathologically elevated. Individuals with lower expression of glucocorticoid receptors in brain regions involved in negative feedback of the stress system are understood to have increased HPA activity both at baseline and during times of stress. Alternatively, higher levels of expression are associated with lower HPA tone. Similarly, if expression of FK506 binding protein 51 (FKBP5, a co-chaperone) is altered, then efficient glucocorticoid inhibition—and thus HPA activity—is disrupted. As a result, a variety of studies have found alterations in glucocorticoid receptor number and sensitivity within the HPA axis in pathological stress states, including PTSD, mood disorders, and anxiety disorders (see Lehrner and Yehuda [2018] and McEwen et al. [2015] for in-depth reviews). Treatment with antidepressants has been shown to restore the function of the negative feedback mechanism.

As described above, the body's stress response is designed to promote survival in the face of sudden, short-term threats. The rapid stress response expects a time-limited threat to briefly activate a behavioral response (fight, flight, freeze, etc.), with a return to baseline once the threat is neutralized. The system is not designed to withstand chronic stress or frequent reexperiencing of significant stress. As such, across the research literature, chronic and early life stress have been repeatedly associated with later development of psychopathology (e.g., Scott et al. 2010).

Childhood Trauma and Abuse

Early life stress—even prenatal exposure—can have significant downstream effects on brain maturation and development, including dysregulation of the HPA axis. Excessive stress can yield negative effects at any time in an individual's life, but the period of childhood carries a higher sensitivity to poor outcomes with stress exposure and is therefore considered a window of vulnerability. This vulnerability comes during a period of distinctly elevated synaptic plasticity and a time of rapid environmental shaping. (When the environment provides positive, nurturing stimuli to scaffold adaptive change, the same time period is called a window of opportunity.)

Traumatic experiences in childhood take a variety of presentations. Physical abuse, sexual abuse, emotional abuse, and neglect are some of the major forms. The ACE studies added several important adverse experiences to this list, such as often feeling unsupported, unimportant, unloved; parents separating/divorcing; witnessing domestic violence; and someone in the house misusing substances, having mental illness, or going to prison. The series of ACE studies (Felitti et al. 1998) showed that first of all, ACEs are incredibly common: half to two-thirds of people filling out the survey experienced at least one ACE. Second, ACEs have an effect on later mental health and physical health, both directly through physiological effects and indirectly through shaping behaviors. Those who experience ACEs are more likely to engage in smoking, misuse of alcohol and substances, and other risky behaviors such as having multiple sexual partners. Third, the effect of childhood adversity is dose dependent: individuals with higher ACE scores (higher levels of early life stress) are more likely to develop not only mental illness including suicidality, but also various pathologies across multiple organ systems, such as diabetes, cardiovascular and pulmonary disease, and cancer.

Studies of long-term effects of early trauma unearth some interesting patterns. Even after controlling for maladaptive coping mechanisms associated with poor health outcomes, such as smoking, individuals with early trauma still have an increased chance of poor health outcomes. These outcomes occur globally in the body, indicating a biological impact that has an organism-wide effect. Neuroanatomical research has demonstrated that early trauma and adversity alter the developmental trajectory in a variety of brain regions, particularly over corticolimbic structures necessary for behavioral and emotional regulation. Research looking to better understand the biological factors driving these changes have uncovered epigenetic mechanisms. Here, we focus on the epigenetic effects of childhood trauma, with emphasis on the glucocorticoid system owing to its relevance in the stress response and its significant representation in the research world.

NR3C1

Factors affecting the expression of the glucocorticoid receptor gene, **nuclear receptor subfamily 3 group C member 1 (NR3C1)**, may have downstream effects on stress response and pathology. A combination of many studies have contributed to this overall understanding. One recent study examined peripheral blood in a clinical population. Wang et al. (2017) found that adults with generalized anxiety disorder displayed increased methylation over a particular *NR3C1* promoter region (exon 1F) compared with control subjects, and the increased methylation was associated with a decrease in expression of *NR3C1* (as measured by a decrease in *NR3C1* mRNA levels). Physiologically, this decrease in expression of *NR3C1* was associated with decreased glucocorticoid responsiveness and dysregulated serum basal cortisol levels. Other studies have shown that methylation changes of *NR3C1* are tied to later pathology, including one prospective study of adolescents. van der Knaap et al. (2015) showed that higher methylation in one region of *NR3C1* (from a peripheral blood sample at age 16) was predictive of later scores on internalizing problems (including depression and anxiety symptoms), as well as lifetime diagnosis of depressive or anxiety disorder. Tyrka et al. (2015) showed that the effect could be seen as early as childhood. The authors examined methylation of the *NR3C1* promoter region (using saliva/buccal cells from children 3–5 years old). They were already able to observe differences in methylation in portions of exon 1 of the promoter region in children with early adversity exposure (maltreatment, stressors, and maltreatment composite).

With an understanding that methylation patterns of *NR3C1* may affect expression, and subsequently correlate with dysfunction of the stress response and development of pathology, it becomes clear that factors affecting methylation patterns of *NR3C1* are relevant to downstream pathology. In their landmark study demonstrating the potential for the environment to influence methylation of this region, Weaver et al. (2004) showed that the epigenome can be affected by early maternal behaviors in rodents. The authors examined maternal behaviors of rats (frequency of licking/grooming and arched-back nursing as opposed to passive nursing) and compared DNA methylation of the promoter region of the glucocorticoid receptor within hippocampal tissue samples. Results were notable in that offspring of mothers demonstrating higher contact through more licking/grooming and nursing showed a distinct pattern of methylation of the promoter region of the glucocorticoid receptor, with associated alterations in histone acetylation, and binding of an additional transcription factor (NGFI-A) as early as the first week of life and persisting into adulthood. Importantly, the group differences were found to reverse with cross-fostering, and all group differences—from DNA methylation and histone acetylation to glucocorticoid receptor expression and hypothalamic-pituitary-adrenal axis (HPA axis) response to stress—disappeared when the rats were infused with a histone deacetylase inhibitor.

In humans, exposure to childhood trauma may have effects on *NR3C1* methylation. McGowan et al. (2009) examined human postmortem hippocampal brain samples, comparing suicide victims who had experienced child abuse, suicide victims who had not experienced child abuse, and control subjects who died suddenly from causes other than suicide. The authors examined expression and methylation of *NR3C1* in hippocampal tissue. *NR3C1* expression was decreased in this region of the brain in suicide victims with a history of childhood abuse compared with control subjects, but not in suicide victims without history of childhood abuse. Levels of *NR3C1* expression corresponded with the methylation status of *NR3C1*, specifically the CpG islands of exon 1F, where a pattern of increased methylation was evident in samples from suicide victims with history of abuse, but not in those without childhood abuse or control subjects.

Methylation of the *NR3C1* promoter region is also associated with a change in HPA axis function in adults with a history of abuse (Tyrka et al. 2012). The authors examined DNA methylation over the *NR3C1* promoter region (including exon 1F) in leukocytes from a peripheral blood sample. Adults answered questions about their trauma history, then completed a dexamethasone suppression/corticotropin-releasing hormone challenge. Participants who experienced early adversity through loss of a parent, maltreatment, or low-quality parenting demonstrated increased methylation over this region. Furthermore, the increased methylation was associated with altered HPA activity, as measured by an attenuated cortisol response in the dexamethasone suppression/corticotropin-releasing hormone challenge. These results may indicate a maladaptive response to chronic stress through a complicated developmental trajectory with early HPA hyperactivation.

Shields et al. (2016) examined methylation from an area called the CpG island shores, regions within 2 kilobases flanking the CpG islands of the promoter where additional functional methylation sites are located. Using blood samples gathered from nearly 300 African American women enrolled in the Black Women's Health Study, the authors examined methylation in a specific area of the CpG shore (similar to FREE1 and FREE2 in *FMR1*; see Chapter 3, "Epigenetics in Neurodevelopmental and Neurodegenerative Disorders") downstream from the *NR3C1* promoter. Methylation status was shown to be associated with abuse in childhood: higher methylation levels were found in participants reporting high frequency of physical abuse relative to women not reporting abuse, with a possible dose-dependent effect. Methylation was also higher in adults reporting a history of sexual abuse, with a significant trend of more severe abuse being linked to higher methylation.

Taken together, these studies show effects of childhood trauma and adversity on *NR3C1*. These effects appear to have negative downstream consequences on HPA axis functioning as well as emergence of pathology. Importantly, this relationship has been found in a variety of sources, including postmortem brain samples, peripheral blood, and buccal cells.

FKBP5

A major regulator of the glucocorticoid signal transduction pathway, FKBP5, is also epigenetically susceptible to stress. As discussed previously in Table 4–1, FKBP5 exercises an overall inhibitory function on glucocorticoid receptor signaling. Expression of *FKBP5* increases with the presence of activated glucocorticoid receptors, which adhere to the glucocorticoid response elements (GREs) of *FKBP5*, stimulating transcription. In this way, *FKBP5* is upregulated by stress. Further, this relationship creates an ultrashort feedback loop: once translated, FKBP5 binds to the glucocorticoid receptor complex, attenuating the effect of the glucocorticoid (Table 4–2) (Matosin et al. 2018).

Activity and expression of *FKBP5* are modulated by several additional factors beyond binding of the glucocorticoid receptor to GREs, including *FKBP5* single-nucleotide polymorphisms (SNPs), environmental stressors, and epigenetic modifications. Epigenetic modifications at the level of the histone include histone H3 lysine 4 trimethylation (H3K4me3), lysine 27 acetylation (H3K27ac), and lysine 36 trimethylation (H3K36me3) (Zannas et al. 2016). It has also been shown that significant stress during certain developmental periods can lead to demethylation of *FKBP5* GREs, as mediated by glucocorticoid receptor activation. This effect is driven in part by exposure to glucocorticoids, as similar patterns of hypomethylation of the *FKBP5* GREs can be produced through early exposure to dexamethasone. Demethylation at these GREs then increases the rate of transcription of the gene when stimulated by an activated glucocorticoid-receptor complex. It is important to note that *FKBP5* variants arising from genetic polymorphisms have varied susceptibility to epigenetic effects (Yeo et al. 2017).

FKBP5 has a variety of alleles which themselves have been associated with differential susceptibility to mental illness, including major depressive disorder (MDD) and PTSD (Klengel et al. 2013). Interestingly, researchers have found that the different alleles show differential susceptibility to epigenetic changes as well. Tozzi et al. (2018) used peripheral blood samples from adults with and without MDD, looking at DNA methylation by allele type (based on specific rs1360780 SNP, which varies as either cytosine, C [low risk], or thymine, T [high risk]), comparing individuals based on childhood trauma. The authors found that individuals with childhood trauma and the higher-risk allele (T) were more likely to show lower methylation of *FKBP5*. The lower methylation patterns were also associated with related gray matter changes in the inferior orbital frontal gyrus and differences in activation patterns during an emotion recognition task.

Table 4–2. *FKBP5* in chronic stress and HPA axis dysregulation

Under normal circumstances, activated glucocorticoid receptors bind to GREs of *FKBP5*, upregulating expression of *FKBP5*.
FKBP5 then downregulates the activity of activated glucocorticoid receptors through an ultrashort negative feedback loop.
Excess glucocorticoid receptor activation during developmentally sensitive time periods leads to demethylation of *FKBP5* GREs, with subsequent increase in the basal expression of *FKBP5*.
Increased basal expression of *FKBP5* has been shown to correlate with decreased response to glucocorticoid presence (i.e., glucocorticoid resistance) via a delay in the negative feedback loop of the HPA axis, resulting in a prolonged cortisol response following stress.
Prolonged cortisol response may further demethylate *FKBP5*, amplifying the circuit and prolonging cortisol response.
In brain regions involved in emotional regulation, these molecular changes could lead to the development of psychiatric disorders.

Note. *FKBP5*=FK506 binding protein 51; GRE=glucocorticoid response element; HPA axis=hypothalamic-pituitary-adrenal axis.
Source. Summary based on Matosin et al. (2018).

It has been argued that the risk genotype itself does not lead to pathology, but rather the risk genotype becomes maladaptive in the presence of childhood trauma. In people carrying the rs1360780-T risk allele and reporting a history of childhood trauma, baseline expression of *FKBP5* is inversely correlated with induction of *FKBP5* expression by dexamethasone administration (Yeo et al. 2017). In other words, individuals with low baseline *FKBP5* expression show larger increases in expression following administration of an exogenous glucocorticoid than do those with high baseline *FKBP5* expression. This relationship suggests a ceiling effect, in which individuals with elevated basal *FKBP5* expression may be more prone to developing a dysregulated stress response owing to reduced responsiveness of FKBP5 to glucocorticoid presence, thus contributing to glucocorticoid resistance. Notably, this relationship does not emerge in individuals carrying the risk allele who do not experience childhood trauma. Furthermore, the authors found a decrease in genome methylation of specific CpG sites in those with trauma history and the risk allele that was not found in those with either no childhood trauma or the protective allele.

FKBP5 expression has been found to be affected by microRNAs (miRNAs) as well. Select miRNAs have been found to regulate *FKBP5*; for example, miRNA-15A and miRNA-511 have both been found to downregulate *FKBP5* expression (Zheng et al. 2016). In mice, chronic stress exposure may cause an increase in miRNA-15A expression in the amygdala, with associated decrease in *FKBP5* expression (Volk et al. 2016). This relationship of stress and miRNA was also found in peripheral blood samples of humans, where miRNA-15A may be elevated in adults who had childhood trauma.

Other Notable Receptors

Additional receptors that may show epigenetic effects from childhood trauma include the opioid receptor, the oxytocin receptor (OXTR), neuropeptide Y, and serotonin transporter SLC6A4, although evidence remains limited. **Glutamate receptor subunit ε-2 (*GRIN2B*)** encodes a subunit of the *N*-methyl-D-aspartate (NMDA) receptor and is susceptible to methylation changes from environmental stressors. Mutations of *GRIN2B* have been associated with a variety of neurodevelopmental and psychiatric disorders. In a longitudinal study, adults provided saliva samples and retrospectively self-reported early adversity (Engdahl et al. 2021). Childhood adversity was defined as having at least two of a list of adverse events before the age of 18, including a parental death, major/severe financial problems, and major/severe disturbances in the family. After controlling for symptoms of depression and alcohol use, authors found a trend of increased methylation of CpG islands of the regulatory region of *GRIN2B* in individuals reporting childhood adversity. This finding, that *GRIN2B* is sensitive to early stressors, builds on prior studies demonstrating effects of in utero exposures to toxins (specifically bisphenol A) on *GRIN2B* methylation (Alavian-Ghavanini et al. 2018).

Another gene studied with regard to childhood trauma is monoamine oxidase A (*MAOA*). Polymorphisms of *MAOA*—the highly expressed long allele and the less efficiently transcribed short allele—have been associated with psychiatric illnesses. Beyond differences in transcription based on alleles, variability in expression has been tied to methylation of this region: higher levels of methylation typically lead to lower levels of MAO enzymatic activity (Shumay et al. 2012). In addition, methylation of *MAOA* is affected by the environment. Over relatively short time scales (on the order of 1 year in adulthood), negative life events may be related to a decrease in methylation of the *MAOA* promoter, whereas recent positive life events are tied to increases in methylation (Domschke et al. 2012). Over a longer time scale, relationships between environmental events and *MAOA* methylation emerge, as demonstrated in a study examining the relationship between types of past abuse, *MAOA* hypermethylation, and *MAOA* genotype in women (Checknita et al. 2018). Study participants completed rating scales on physical abuse from parents and sexual abuse from any person in authority. DNA samples were extracted from saliva and genotyped for the short versus long allele of *MAOA*. Methylation was then analyzed specifically in the CpG islands of the promoter region of *MAOA*. The results showed a significant trend of methylation differences in those who experienced physical abuse compared with those who did not, and an even more robust trend in the sexual abuse group compared with never-abused participants. This finding of differential methylation based on type of abuse is consistent with other studies that have shown the quantitative effects of trauma—a higher number of ACEs related to more negative outcomes—and also qualitative differences in outcomes depending on the type of trauma experienced.

Studies using modern, epigenomewide DNA methylation microarrays have provided a glimpse of larger patterns of epigenetic markings of trauma, outside of the single-gene approaches discussed here. Using a consortium of cohorts with a combined N=1896, Smith et al. (2020) used the Illumina Infinium HumanMethylation450 BeadChip (450,000 sites) to find reduced methylation of the **aryl hydrocarbon receptor repressor (*AHRR*)** gene in individuals with PTSD compared with unaffected trauma-exposed control subjects. *AHRR* has a well-established link to smoking (as discussed in Chapter 5, "Epigenetics of Lifestyle and Aging") and plays a role in immune function, and the authors provided evidence that the relationship of reduced *AHRR* methylation at four CpG sites in PTSD was independent of smoking effects. A study that examined DNA methylation using the Illumina EPIC BeadChip (850,000 sites) in blood and brain samples of U.S. veterans replicated the significant association with *AHRR*, above and beyond its well-established link to smoking, while highlighting an association with the G0/G1 switch 2 (*GoS2*) gene, which has been tied to a number of processes including lipid metabolism, cell communication, and cell death (Logue et al. 2020). Other studies using methylation microarrays have found further associations of reduced methylation in markers associated with the immune system (Uddin et al. 2010). Additionally, there is some evidence of differences in DNA methylation enrichment patterns across the genome of individuals with PTSD, depending on whether they experienced abuse in childhood (Mehta et al. 2013).

Transgenerational Trauma

The transmission of trauma experience from parent to future generations is often depicted as a cycle: individuals who experience abuse and neglect in childhood grow up to become adults who are more likely to subject their own offspring to abuse and neglect. This cycle of intergenerational or transgenerational trauma may seem simple on the surface, but the driving mechanisms are complex. In one respect, abuse and neglect modeled by the parent may become learned behaviors that the child then acts out in adulthood. Additionally, individuals with their own exposures to early childhood adversity are more likely to develop functional changes or "scars" in the brain, especially in circuits essential for emotional control, inhibition, learning, and memory functions, increasing the risk of perpetuating abuse. These effects are modulated in part through GxE interactions. As such, an adult who has experienced early childhood adversity has a higher risk of displaying abusive, neglectful, or otherwise dysfunctional behaviors toward the next generation, creating adverse experiences with subsequent neurobehavioral sequelae.

Epigenetics adds another layer to understanding the cycle of trauma within a family. Epigenetic changes can be temporary or they can be long-lasting, even to the point that they can be transmitted to progeny. Typically, during the process of forming gametes and embryos, there is a great degree of chromatin restructuring, demethylation, and other erasing of epigenetic marks; however, some marks persist despite this opportunity to reset. For this reason, the toxic effects of trauma can transcend one's own lifetime, with "epigenetic scars" being passed along to future generations, independent of behaviors of the parent. In other words, individuals may carry the epigenetic marks of trauma from a prior generation even if they have not experienced or witnessed trauma firsthand. The efforts to characterize these forms of epigenetic inheritance are discussed here.

In the literature, a variety of terms refer to effects of stress passed on from prior generations, and the differences are worth delineating. **Preconception stress** comes from the rodent-model literature and refers specifically to stressful experiences occurring within a short window of time just before conception. In rats, this is studied over a matter of weeks, and even stress experienced in this brief period before conception can have consequences on brain structure, HPA function, and behavior (Gröger et al. 2016). Stress occurring after conception but before birth is termed **gestational stress** or **prenatal stress** and has been found to strongly impact later behaviors, such as those associated with depression and anxiety, and to affect development of neural structures across frontal and limbic regions. Outside this perinatal window, the distinction between **intergenerational** and **transgenerational transmission** is based on whether offspring come from gametes formed before or after trauma exposure, respectively (see Lehrner and Yehuda [2018] for more detail), which may become important when approaching some literature but is not further distinguished here. As a general notion, intergenerational and transgenerational (or even multigenerational) trauma refers to the effects of a trauma from long before conception being transmitted to an individual, and perhaps even to later generations.

Thus far, the most robust data on transgenerational effects of trauma come from studies on shared cultural trauma. Yehuda et al. (2016) examined CpG methylation of *FKBP5* in male and female Holocaust survivors and their offspring, compared with matched unexposed control subjects. Distinct methylation patterns of *FKBP5* coupled with differences in basal cortisol levels emerged in both the survivors and their offspring. These similarities in methylation patterns and glucocorticoid function that Holocaust survivors shared with their offspring were independent of the offspring's own trauma exposure or psychopathology. Lehrner and Yehuda (2018) later expanded on the effects of the Holocaust, referring to it as a "case study of cultural trauma" and sharing a litany of references to the intergenerational impacts of other genocides and epic cultural traumas such as colonization, slavery, and war. Although they focus on significant stressors occurring at the cultural level, many of their statements can be applied to epigenetic transmission of other significant traumas. Accordingly, Grasso et al. (2020) examined intergenerational epigenetic effects of individual adversity and trauma on methylation of *FKBP5*, demonstrating that history of ACEs in mothers may be tied to allele-specific epigenetic patterns in infants at birth.

In Utero Stress Exposure

Conversations about the transgenerational effects of stress and trauma frequently include toxic exposures in the womb. The epigenetic effects of in utero exposure can be particularly far-reaching, considering that oogenesis in females begins during fetal development. By the time a girl is born, her ovaries already contain all her ova, which will remain dormant until she becomes fertile and ovulation begins. Therefore, in the same moments, any effects from toxic physiological or environmental exposures that a pregnant mother experiences may impact her own epigenome, the epigenome of her developing daughter, and the epigenome of the gamete destined to be fertilized and become her grandchild.

Epigenetic effects of in utero exposures have been found across a variety of genes and mechanisms. As discussed above, miRNAs play a vital role in neurogenesis, synaptogenesis, neural transmission, neural plasticity, and neurodegeneration. Changes to the function of miRNAs occur following stress responses. As with other epigenetic changes, miRNAs show alteration after extreme stress and contribute to subsequent pathological neural function. This has been observed at the fundamental level of the neurons themselves, and it has also been shown that stress exposure can affect miRNA expression in a brain region–specific manner, notably affecting the frontal cortex and hippocampus. As such, research has shown that prenatal exposure to several different types of stress, including maternal anxiety, toxin exposure, and infection, can affect a variety of miRNAs with the potential to modulate the expression of innumerable genes (see Hollins and Cairns [2016] for a review). These epigenetic effects may then contribute to alterations in brain development, with subsequent pathology including developmental disorders (e.g., autism spectrum disorder and ADHD) and later increased risk for mood, anxiety, and psychotic disorder emergence.

Research has also shown effects of in utero exposure on methylation patterns of the epigenome. The relationship between in utero stress exposure and epigenetic effects of glucocorticoid receptor components was studied in placentas of mothers at term. Ratings of perceived stress were related to elevations in promoter methylation of both *FKBP5* and the 11β-hydroxysteroid dehydrogenase gene, a relationship tied functionally to relatively lower recordings of fetal central nervous system development (Monk et al. 2016). In another study, mothers exposed to intimate partner violence while pregnant did not show changes to methylation patterns of the glucocorticoid receptor, but their offspring did show changes into adolescence (Radtke et al. 2011). Additional studies have demonstrated epigenetic effects of in utero stress on the dopamine (D2) receptor, *BDNF*, and *OXTR*.

The biological effects of trauma, even trauma before birth or conception, can paint a rather bleak portrait of posttrauma development. However, there are two points of hope. First, not all people who experience these traumas develop pathological responses. Second, the epigenome is in a constant, dynamic state of change, frequently updating itself to prepare optimally for the predicted future environment. Therefore, it seems possible to at least partially reverse the epigenetic scars from trauma through interventions. These optimistic viewpoints are the focus of the next section.

Resilience

Defining Resilience

Resilience has had many definitions across research but may be thought of generally as a buffer for the risk of developing pathological responses to adverse events. Resilience is incredibly complex and may be better understood as "stress armor," forged from biopsychosocial materials, as it contains elements across a variety of interacting levels. As Masten (2011) eloquently defined, resilience is "the capacity of a dynamic system to withstand or recover from significant challenges that threaten its stability, viability, or development." Biologically, we can think in terms of neurophysiology, breaking concepts down into genetic and epigenetic effects—as discussed here—but it is important to be aware of the other moderators of resilience. Psychologically, resilience is understood in terms of traits such as temperament and grit, general self-efficacy, and ways of thinking such as cognitive reappraisals, as well as other positive cognitive emotion regulation strategies or coping mechanisms an individual may enact. Also, resilience is socially influenced by availability of support from one's culture, neighborhood, peer groups, and family. Considering this short, nonexclusive list of components, it becomes clear that in many ways resilience is actually an active adaptability process. It may be argued that a big component of mental health treatment is instilling resilience, reducing symptom burden, educating, teaching coping mechanisms, and promoting a healthy lifestyle, all of which aim to give the patient a better chance at adaptively responding to future stressors.

An alternative, very common way of defining resilience is as the opposite of stress vulnerability. While this definition may be entirely valid, and perhaps more attractive in its simplicity, it is incomplete. Studies using this oversimplification may highlight the absence of risk factors rather than the presence of protective factors to describe resilience. As a result, many studies on resilience may in fact be focusing on the factors that increase vulnerability to stress later in life, and many publications purporting to explore improving mechanisms of resilience are actually examining the prevention of trauma. When it comes to interventions, both prevention of risk factors and promotion of protective factors are crucial. It is therefore important in dissecting the literature to get a sense of how resilience is being operationalized. Of course, prevention of childhood trauma and stress is at the forefront of our efforts, but the question remains: for children exposed to these traumas, are there protective factors, or even interventions, that may enhance resilience at the biological level? Many studies have shown epigenetic differences between resilient individuals and nonresilient individuals; however, it is difficult to say whether the epigenetic differences initially facilitated the resilience or resulted from it. Here, we focus on epigenetic mechanisms related to resilience, emphasizing ones that appear responsive to intervention.

Epigenetics of Resilience

The biological and neurological underpinnings of resilience are notably complex (see Osório et al. [2017] for a review). Whereas childhood has been considered a window of vulnerability, during which an insult may drastically affect one's developmental trajectory, Andersen (2003) inserted some optimism into this paradigm by describing the timing of plasticity of the child's brain rather as a window of opportunity. For example, having close, comforting, supportive relationships during childhood is associated with improved developmental trajectories through to adulthood, buffering the consequences of toxic stress (Chen et al. 2017). This window of opportunity never closes completely, as opportunities to build resilience do not end in childhood. Treatment of psychopathology often involves interventions that affect the brain, ultimately harnessing its plasticity, whether treatment be pharmaceutical or nonpharmaceutical (McEwen 2016).

One study examining how DNA methylation patterns may relate to resilience in childhood specifically examined *OXTR* (Milaniak et al. 2017). The authors found that in children prenatally exposed to adversity, a methylation pattern of *OXTR* present in cord blood at time of birth was associated with differences in mother-reported conduct problems later on. Specifically, results suggested that higher levels of *OXTR* methylation at birth are related to lower conduct problem scores in middle childhood. It is unclear whether this methylation difference would lead to higher or lower expression of *OXTR*, as other studies have shown conflicting relationships between methylation and higher or lower circulating oxytocin levels.

Some studies have examined the effects of interventions on reducing the effects of trauma. In one study of rodents, placing maternal and paternal rats into a positively enriched environment for 4 weeks before mating evoked patterns of decreased methylation across the genome of the progeny (as measured in hippocampal and frontal cortex tissue), accompanied by observed benefits in neurodevelopmental trajectory and behavior (Mychasiuk et al. 2012). In mice, it has been further shown that enrichment of the father's environment before conception can buffer transgenerational trauma, resetting some of the aberrant DNA methylation of the glucocorticoid receptor gene, with subsequently improved glucocorticoid receptor expression and reduced behavioral symptoms of trauma in the offspring (Gapp et al. 2016).

Interventions in clinical samples have also been promising. One study examined *NR3C1* and *FKBP5* in children and adolescents who received cognitive-behavioral therapy for anxiety (Roberts et al. 2015). No genetic or epigenetic biomarker was found to predict who would respond positively to therapy. However, the authors did find a relationship between change in genome methylation and treatment response that followed an allele-specific methylation pattern. Children and adolescents carrying the *FKBP5* risk alleles accompanied by a decrease in percentage of DNA methylation after therapy were more likely to experience greater reduction in symptom severity following therapy. There was no relationship of methylation changes relative to treatment response for *NR3C1* or nonrisk *FKBP5* allele carriers.

Another important study examined epigenetic effects of the Nurse-Family Partnership project, which is a longitudinal, randomized intervention (O'Donnell et al. 2018). The intervention identifies mothers at high risk for displaying abusive parenting practices and schedules regular nurse visits during prenatal and early development that focus on the mother-child interaction and health of the mother. This program has been found to reduce the occurrence of child abuse and neglect, with subsequent benefits over a variety of neurodevelopmental outcomes. In this particular study, a significant difference in DNA methylation was observed at 27 years of age (25 years after conclusion of intervention) in offspring of mothers who completed the intervention program compared with control subjects. The differences in DNA methylation were found across the genome but also observed in particular loci including *NR3C1*. Therefore, this intervention designed to reduce childhood adversity led to benefits in adulthood accompanied by sustained differences in DNA methylation across the genome, including regions specifically relevant to the stress response. Effects remained significant even after controlling for additional risky behaviors such as smoking, which can affect the epigenome. This intervention also suggests that early psychosocial intervention with support for mothers and their families can reduce childhood trauma, promote resilience, and improve risk factors of offspring into adulthood, actively moving toward breaking the cycle of violence.

At the time of this writing, a limited number of studies have examined the role of histone methylation and acetylation in experience of trauma; some studies in rodents have demonstrated a role of histone deacetylases in both the fear memory process and the development of resilience. Histone modification therefore is a research area of expected growth. Changes in miRNAs have also been associated with trauma and resilience. Research in this field continues to grow, but only a few select forms of miRNA have been found to play a role in trauma response and resilience, in particular as they relate to development of depression (see Lopizzo et al. [2019] for a review). Further, miRNAs have been shown to relate to

treatment response of antidepressants. Finally, miRNAs are being investigated as a potential therapy in the form of medication that acts by RNA
interference, decreasing production of problematic proteins. Currently
only one such RNA-interfering pharmacotherapy has approval from the
FDA for a specific form of hereditary amyloidosis, but this is a promising
therapeutic option for the future.

As a final caution in assessing trauma and resilience, recent studies
have examined how resilience may be only "skin deep," calling into question the best definition of resilience. For instance, some individuals respond to early adversity with self-discipline and hard work, showing
success academically and professionally while exhibiting strong self-
esteem. Despite this outward appearance of psychosocial resilience, be-
neath the surface are biological processes that reflect continuation of a
dysregulated stress response and subsequent medical comorbidities
(Brody et al. 2016). This phenomenon, skin-deep resilience, provides an
additional confounding factor for the role of biological processes—possibly including epigenetics—in which a well-adjusted, apparently resilient
individual may share biological markings and pathological sequelae of a
less successful, less psychologically or socially resilient peer with similar
trauma experience.

Considerations for Approaching Current Literature

An important distinction is the difference between trauma vulnerability
and resilience. As discussed above, in trauma and resilience research, the
operational definitions of trauma and trauma vulnerability are relatively
simple. Resilience, on the other hand, is much more complex, as it incor-
porates the limitation of vulnerabilities and the presence of strengths to
buffer effects of adversity. One difficulty is deciding whether a study that
purports to discuss resilience is actually doing so, or whether it is actually
discussing the prevention of trauma and trauma vulnerability. Of course,
trauma prevention is essential, but resilience is not simply trauma prevention. Consumers of research must remain vigilant in perusing works
on "resilience" that may be better defined as works on trauma vulnerability prevention.

Another detail of crucial importance in studies of individuals exposed
to trauma is the effect of smoking. As will be discussed further in Chapter
5, "Epigenetics of Lifestyle and Aging," smoking carries widespread effects
across the epigenome. Early trauma and ACEs are related to negative outcomes and negative health behaviors, including elevated risk of smoking.

It is therefore essential for study designs to control for negative health behaviors such as smoking, because such behaviors may act as mediators or moderators of clinical and physiological outcomes, especially in the case of smoking and early childhood adversity (Sugden et al. 2019).

The future of epigenetics in trauma and resilience is promising. Although this research niche is in its early stages, it is supported by the substantive, foundational work of the developmental effects of trauma and resilience. Further research on physiology, including interesting work regarding the epigenetic effects on permeability of the blood–brain barrier (Dudek et al. 2020), may carve new avenues for trauma and resilience research as well. Future directions include isolating epigenetic markers of the resilient phenotype, trauma vulnerability risks, and treatment response following interventions. Perhaps clinical practice will find an application of epigenetics in predicting response to therapeutic modalities when devising treatment plans.

Conclusion

A striking proportion of individuals face adversity throughout life. This adversity may translate into epigenetic changes, which may then drive changes in gene expression. As discussed in this chapter, epigenetic effects can stem from childhood trauma; earlier toxic exposures in utero; or even earlier events before conception. The consequent epigenetic marks may then be passed through reproduction to future generations.

However, not all individuals subjected to stress and trauma, either pre- or postconception, develop maladaptive physiological or behavioral effects. This dynamic ability to endure stress and trauma, known as resilience (which includes factors that help buffer trauma vulnerability), has become its own focus of research. Some studies have demonstrated that resilient individuals carry their own biological signatures; importantly, interventions to enhance resilience have been found to yield biological effects down to the epigenome. Therefore, although the profound developmental effects of trauma may seem unrelenting, perpetuating abuse and trauma across generations, there is hope in the power of supportive people, enriched environments, and early interventions for at-risk families to undo some of these effects of adversity.

KEY POINTS

- Mental illness can be a consequence of early life adversity.
- Low to moderate levels of stress are not pathological; in fact, they may play a role in successful development and resilience forma-

tion. Stress that is excessive in magnitude or frequency can bring about maladaptive change in physiological and behavioral response systems. Some individuals are more predisposed to developing pathological stress responses.

- Individuals who are exposed to toxic stress may exhibit changes in brain circuitry that can lead to dysfunction in emotion regulation, cognition, and behaviors, with subsequently increased risk of developing physical and mental illness. Research into the effects of environmental stress has uncovered the presence of complex epigenetic mechanisms that may play a role in these effects on human physiology and disease.

- The physiology of the stress response involves the hypothalamic-pituitary-adrenal axis (HPA axis) and corticolimbic pathways, both of which are rich in glucocorticoid receptors. The function of glucocorticoid receptors and chaperones, including FK506 binding protein 51 (FKBP5), is crucial for adequate inhibition of the stress response. Disruption to the function of glucocorticoid receptors and FKBP5 has been tied to chronic stress and development of pathology.

- Early environment, particularly childhood trauma and adversity, produces epigenetic effects around *NR3C1* that affect expression. These changes in expression of glucocorticoid receptors are associated with effects on HPA axis functioning, including cortisol levels and glucocorticoid sensitivity, as well as later development of mood and anxiety symptoms.

- FKBP5 is an important regulator of the glucocorticoid receptor, playing a predominantly inhibitory role in glucocorticoid effects. A variety of epigenetic effects—including methylation changes in glucocorticoid response elements (GREs), histone modification, and miRNA induction—emerge from childhood trauma and contribute to subsequent stress response disruption.

- Transgenerational trauma occurs through a variety of mechanisms, including epigenetics. People with a history of significant trauma may produce children who share epigenetic marks of these traumas, even in the absence of any firsthand trauma experience in the child.

- In utero, the epigenome of the fetus is susceptible to environmental stress exposures. The epigenome within gametes of the fetus may also be affected, opening the possibility for effects to carry into the next generation.

- Childhood is considered a window of vulnerability because of the higher sensitivity to poor outcomes with stress exposure during this time. This vulnerability comes during a period of distinctly elevated synaptic plasticity. It is important to note that this is a time of rapid environmental shaping, so when the environment provides positive, nurturing stimuli to scaffold adaptive change, then we refer to this same time period as a window of opportunity.

- Resilience is complex and pertains to more than the absence of stress vulnerability. Interventions devised to enhance resilience are limited in number, but some studies have shown benefits from these interventions that are associated with changes of the epigenome.

Study Questions

1. Which hormone has a predominantly inhibitory role on the HPA axis?

   A. Corticotropin-releasing hormone (CRH)
   B. Arginine vasopressin (AVP)
   C. Adrenocorticotropic hormone (ACTH)
   D. Cortisol

   Best answer: D

   Explanation: CRH, AVP, ACTH, and cortisol are essential hormones of the HPA axis. Both CRH (answer A) and AVP (answer B) are released by the hypothalamus and stimulate the pituitary gland to release ACTH. ACTH (answer C) stimulates the adrenal cortex, releasing cortisol. Cortisol (answer D) then inhibits HPA activity through a negative feedback mechanism by activating glucocorticoid receptors of the hypothalamus and pituitary.

2. Which of the following is true about glucocorticoid receptors?

   A. A majority of glucocorticoid receptors are located in the cell membrane to facilitate transport of cortisol into the cell.
   B. Glucocorticoid receptors contain GREs, to which chaperones such as FKBP5 bind.
   C. An activated glucocorticoid receptor has different effects inside and outside the nucleus.
   D. FKBP5 enhances the activity of glucocorticoid receptors.

Best answer: C

Explanation: Activated glucocorticoid receptors have genomic effects inside the nucleus and nongenomic effects outside the nucleus (answer C). Inside the nucleus, they can bind to DNA to increase or decrease transcription of certain genes. Outside the nucleus, they may interact with a variety of other cell pathways. Cortisol is nonpolar and passes freely across the cell membrane (eliminating answer A). Glucocorticoid receptors are nuclear receptors, predominantly in the cytosol, and interact with cortisol after it has moved into the cell. GREs (answer B) are found in the promoter regions of genes that are regulated by glucocorticoids. GREs are sites on the genome where the activated glucocorticoid receptor attaches to allow regulation of transcription. FKBP5 (answer D) is a chaperone that interacts with the glucocorticoid receptor complex, typically inhibiting it.

3.   When do epigenetic effects of childhood adversity begin to emerge?

A. Childhood
B. Adolescence
C. Early adulthood
D. Late adulthood

Best answer: A

Explanation: Studies have found changes to methylation of *NR3C1* related to childhood adversity across all age groups. One study discussed in this chapter found differences in methylation patterns of *NR3C1* as early as age 3–5 years (answer A).

4.   What effects can childhood adversity have on the glucocorticoid receptor gene (*NR3C1*) and function?

A. Effects on *NR3C1* methylation but not expression, HPA function, or anxiety symptoms.
B. Effects on *NR3C1* methylation and expression, but not HPA function or anxiety symptoms.
C. Effects on *NR3C1* methylation, expression, and HPA function, but not anxiety symptoms.
D. Effects on *NR3C1* methylation, expression, HPA function, and anxiety symptoms.

Best answer: D

Explanation: Multiple studies have demonstrated that childhood trauma and adversity can lead to changes to the methylation pattern of *NR3C1*, typically showing an increase in methylation of exons in the promoter region (answer A). These epigenetic changes are associated with changes to expression of *NR3C1* (answer B) and downstream effects on HPA activity as observed through changes to basal cortisol levels as well as glucocorticoid sensitivity (answer C). Additional studies have also demonstrated that these effects are tied to development of pathology, including later mood and anxiety symptom expression (answer D).

5.   Which of the following genes has robust data supporting an allele-dependent epigenetic effect of childhood trauma?

A. Glucocorticoid receptor (*NR3C1*)
B. FK506 binding protein 51 (*FKBP5*)
C. Glutamate receptor subunit ε-2 (*GRIN2B*)
D. Oxytocin receptor (*OXTR*)

Best answer: B

Explanation: Different alleles of *FKBP5* show differential susceptibility to epigenetic changes (answer B). The identified rs1360780 SNP varies as either cytosine, C (low risk), or thymine, T (high risk). Those with the T allele are more likely to show significant epigenetic effects following childhood trauma than those without childhood trauma or the risk allele. Decreases in genome methylation of specific CpG sites in those with trauma history and the risk allele are not present in those with either no childhood trauma or the protective allele. Currently, there is no evidence for allele-dependent epigenetic effects of childhood trauma in *NR3C1* (answer A), *GRIN2B* (answer C), or *OXTR* (answer D).

6.   What happens to epigenetic marks during reproduction?

A. During gametogenesis, all epigenetic marks are erased.
B. Some epigenetic marks are transmitted to the offspring.
C. Some epigenetic marks from the mother are transmitted to the offspring, but not from the father.
D. The majority of epigenetic marks are transmitted to the offspring.

Best answer: B

Explanation: During gametogenesis and embryogenesis, epigenetic marks (DNA methylation, histone acetylation/methylation, etc.) are erased to a large degree (contradicting answer D), offering a chance for some resetting. This is not the case for all epigenetic marks, however (answer A), as some marks persist. In particular, significant traumatic experiences appear to cause epigenetic changes that may be transferred to future generations, contributing mechanistically to transgenerational trauma (answer B). A study including both male and female Holocaust survivors demonstrated a shared methylation pattern with offspring (contradicting answer C).

7.   Which of the following statements regarding resilience is false?

   A. Neurologically, resilience can be fostered in any age group, not just childhood.
   B. Enriching experiences can undo aberrant DNA methylation patterns of progeny.
   C. Only prevention of trauma has been found to enhance the epigenome.
   D. Although individuals may appear resilient and successful, they may carry physiological effects of early trauma.

Best answer: C

Explanation: Prevention of trauma is important, but it is not the only means to bolster resilience and elicit epigenetic benefits (thus answer C is the false one). From a neurological perspective, childhood presents a window of opportunity (or vulnerability), but the brain maintains some plasticity through to later ages, allowing for continued fostering of resilience (supporting answer A). In studies of rodents, preconception enrichment led to the resetting of epigenetic markings of transgenerational trauma in progeny (supporting answer B). The concept of skin-deep resilience illustrates how individuals with trauma history may take on a phenotype of strong self-esteem and achievement in their social context but continue to carry elevated risks of various pathology, similar to less-resilient-appearing trauma-exposed peers (supporting answer D).

References

Alavian-Ghavanini A, Lin PI, Lind PM, et al: Prenatal bisphenol A exposure is linked to epigenetic changes in glutamate receptor subunit gene Grin2b in female rats and humans. Sci Rep 8(1):11315, 2018 30054528

Andersen SL: Trajectories of brain development: point of vulnerability or window of opportunity? Neurosci Biobehav Rev 27(1–2):3–18, 2003 12732219

Averill LA, Averill CL, Kelmendi B, et al: Stress response modulation underlying the psychobiology of resilience. Curr Psychiatry Rep 20(4):27, 2018 29594808

Broadhurst PL: Emotionality and the Yerkes-Dodson law. J Exp Psychol 54(5):345–352, 1957 13481281

Brody GH, Yu T, Miller GE, Chen E: Resilience in adolescence, health, and psychosocial outcomes. Pediatrics 138(6):e20161042, 2016 27940681

Checknita D, Ekström TJ, Comasco E, et al: Associations of monoamine oxidase A gene first exon methylation with sexual abuse and current depression in women. J Neural Transm (Vienna) 125(7):1053–1064, 2018 29600412

Chen E, Brody GH, Miller GE: Childhood close family relationships and health. Am Psychol 72(6):555–566, 2017 28880102

Domschke K, Tidow N, Kuithan H, et al: Monoamine oxidase A gene DNA hypomethylation—a risk factor for panic disorder? Int J Neuropsychopharmacol 15(9):1217–1228, 2012 22436428

Dudek KA, Dion-Albert L, Lebel M, et al: Molecular adaptations of the blood-brain barrier promote stress resilience vs. depression. Proc Natl Acad Sci USA 117(6):3326–3336, 2020

Engdahl E, Alavian-Ghavanini A, Forsell Y, et al: Childhood adversity increases methylation in the GRIN2B gene. J Psychiatr Res 132:38–43, 2021 33038564

Feder A, Nestler EJ, Charney DS: Psychobiology and molecular genetics of resilience. Nat Rev Neurosci 10(6):446–457, 2009 19455174

Felitti VJ, Anda RF, Nordenberg D, et al: Relationship of childhood abuse and household dysfunction to many of the leading causes of death in adults. The Adverse Childhood Experiences (ACE) Study. Am J Prev Med 14(4):245–258, 1998 9635069

Gapp K, Bohacek J, Grossmann J, et al: Potential of environmental enrichment to prevent transgenerational effects of paternal trauma. Neuropsychopharmacology 41(11):2749–2758, 2016 27277118

Grasso DJ, Drury S, Briggs-Gowan M, et al: Adverse childhood experiences, posttraumatic stress, and FKBP5 methylation patterns in postpartum women and their newborn infants. Psychoneuroendocrinology 114:104604, 2020 32109789

Green JG, McLaughlin KA, Berglund PA, et al: Childhood adversities and adult psychiatric disorders in the national comorbidity survey replication I: associations with first onset of DSM-IV disorders. Arch Gen Psychiatry 67(2):113–123, 2010 20124111

Gröger N, Matas E, Gos T, et al: The transgenerational transmission of childhood adversity: behavioral, cellular, and epigenetic correlates. J Neural Transm (Vienna) 123(9):1037–1052, 2016 27169537

Hollins SL, Cairns MJ: MicroRNA: small RNA mediators of the brain's genomic response to environmental stress. Prog Neurobiol 143:61–81, 2016 27317386

Jankord R, Herman JP: Limbic regulation of hypothalamo-pituitary-adrenocortical function during acute and chronic stress. Ann N Y Acad Sci 1148:64–73, 2008 19120092

Klengel T, Mehta D, Anacker C, et al: Allele-specific FKBP5 DNA demethylation mediates gene-childhood trauma interactions. Nat Neurosci 16(1):33–41, 2013 23201972

Lehrner A, Yehuda R: Cultural trauma and epigenetic inheritance. Dev Psychopathol 30(5):1763–1777, 2018 30261943

Logue MW, Miller MW, Wolf EJ, et al: An epigenome-wide association study of posttraumatic stress disorder in US veterans implicates several new DNA methylation loci. Clin Epigenet 12(1):65, 2020

Lopizzo N, Zonca V, Cattane N, et al: miRNAs in depression vulnerability and resilience: novel targets for preventive strategies. J Neural Transm (Vienna) 126(9):1241–1258, 2019 31350592

Masten AS: Resilience in children threatened by extreme adversity: frameworks for research, practice, and translational synergy. Dev Psychopathol 23(2):493–506, 2011 23786691

Matosin N, Halldorsdottir T, Binder EB: Understanding the molecular mechanisms underpinning gene by environment interactions in psychiatric disorders: the FKBP5 model. Biol Psychiatry 83(10):821–830, 2018 29573791

McEwen BS: In pursuit of resilience: stress, epigenetics, and brain plasticity. Ann N Y Acad Sci 1373(1):56–64, 2016

McEwen BS, Bowles NP, Gray JD, et al: Mechanisms of stress in the brain. Nat Neurosci 18(10):1353–1363, 2015 26404710

McGowan PO, Sasaki A, D'Alessio AC, et al: Epigenetic regulation of the glucocorticoid receptor in human brain associates with childhood abuse. Nat Neurosci 12(3):342–348, 2009 19234457

Mehta D, Klengel T, Conneely KN, et al: Childhood maltreatment is associated with distinct genomic and epigenetic profiles in posttraumatic stress disorder. Proc Natl Acad Sci USA 110(20):8302–8307, 2013

Milaniak I, Cecil CAM, Barker ED, et al: Variation in DNA methylation of the oxytocin receptor gene predicts children's resilience to prenatal stress. Dev Psychopathol 29(5):1663–1674, 2017 29162179

Monk C, Feng T, Lee S, et al: Distress during pregnancy: epigenetic regulation of placenta glucocorticoid-related genes and fetal neurobehavior. Am J Psychiatry 173(7):705–713, 2016 27013342

Mychasiuk R, Zahir S, Schmold N, et al: Parental enrichment and offspring development: modifications to brain, behavior and the epigenome. Behav Brain Res 228(2):294–298, 2012 22173001

Nicolaides NC, Kyratzi E, Lamprokostopoulou A, et al: Stress, the stress system and the role of glucocorticoids. Neuroimmunomodulation 22(1–2):6–19, 2015 25227402

O'Donnell KJ, Chen L, MacIsaac JL, et al: DNA methylome variation in a perinatal nurse-visitation program that reduces child maltreatment: a 27-year follow-up. Transl Psychiatry 8(1):15, 2018 29317599

Osório C, Probert T, Jones E, et al: Adapting to stress: understanding the neurobiology of resilience. Behav Med 43(4):307–322, 2017 27100966

Radtke KM, Ruf M, Gunter HM, et al: Transgenerational impact of intimate partner violence on methylation in the promoter of the glucocorticoid receptor. Transl Psychiatry 1(7):e21, 2011 22832523

Roberts S, Keers R, Lester KJ, et al: HPA axis related genes and response to psychological therapies: genetics and epigenetics. Depress Anxiety 32(12):861–870, 2015 26647360

Schiele MA, Domschke K: Epigenetics at the crossroads between genes, environment and resilience in anxiety disorders. Genes Brain Behav 17(3):e12423, 2018 28873274

Scott KM, Smith DR, Ellis PM: Prospectively ascertained child maltreatment and its association with DSM-IV mental disorders in young adults. Arch Gen Psychiatry 67(7):712–719, 2010 20603452

Shields AE, Wise LA, Ruiz-Narvaez EA, et al: Childhood abuse, promoter methylation of leukocyte NR3C1 and the potential modifying effect of emotional support. Epigenomics 8(11):1507–1517, 2016 27620456

Shumay E, Logan J, Volkow ND, Fowler JS: Evidence that the methylation state of the monoamine oxidase A (MAOA) gene predicts brain activity of MAO A enzyme in healthy men. Epigenetics 7(10):1151–1160, 2012 22948232

Smith AK, Ratanatharathorn A, Maihofer AX, et al: Epigenome-wide meta-analysis of PTSD across 10 military and civilian cohorts identifies methylation changes in AHRR. Nat Commun 11(1):5965, 2020

Sugden K, Hannon EJ, Arseneault L, et al: Establishing a generalized polyepigenetic biomarker for tobacco smoking. Transl Psychiatry 9(1):92, 2019 30770782

Tozzi L, Farrell C, Booij L, et al: Epigenetic changes of FKBP5 as a link connecting genetic and environmental risk factors with structural and functional brain changes in major depression. Neuropsychopharmacology 43(5):1138–1145, 2018 29182159

Tyrka AR, Price LH, Marsit C, et al: Childhood adversity and epigenetic modulation of the leukocyte glucocorticoid receptor: preliminary findings in healthy adults. PLoS One 7(1):e30148, 2012 22295073

Tyrka AR, Parade SH, Eslinger NM, et al: Methylation of exons 1D, 1F, and 1H of the glucocorticoid receptor gene promoter and exposure to adversity in preschool-aged children. Dev Psychopathol 27(2):577–585, 2015 25997773

Uddin M, Aiello AE, Wildman DE, et al: Epigenetic and immune function profiles associated with posttraumatic stress disorder. Proc Natl Acad Sci USA 107(20):9470–9475, 2010

van der Knaap LJ, van Oort FVA, Verhulst FC, et al: Methylation of NR3C1 and SLC6A4 and internalizing problems. The TRAILS study. J Affect Disord 180:97–103, 2015 25889020

Volk N, Pape JC, Engel M, et al: Amygdalar microRNA-15a is essential for coping with chronic stress. Cell Rep 17(7):1882–1891, 2016 27829158

Wang W, Feng J, Ji C, et al: Increased methylation of glucocorticoid receptor gene promoter 1F in peripheral blood of patients with generalized anxiety disorder. J Psychiatr Res 91:18–25, 2017 28292649

Weaver ICG, Cervoni N, Champagne FA, et al: Epigenetic programming by maternal behavior. Nat Neurosci 7(8):847–854, 2004 15220929

Yehuda R, Daskalakis NP, Bierer LM, et al: Holocaust exposure induced intergenerational effects on FKBP5 methylation. Biol Psychiatry 80(5):372–380, 2016 26410355

Yeo S, Enoch MA, Gorodetsky E, et al: The influence of FKBP5 genotype on expression of FKBP5 and other glucocorticoid-regulated genes, dependent on trauma exposure. Genes Brain Behav 16(2):223–232, 2017 27648526

Zannas AS, Wiechmann T, Gassen NC, Binder EB: Gene-stress-epigenetic regulation of FKBP5: clinical and translational implications. Neuropsychopharmacology 41(1):261–274, 2016 26250598

Zheng D, Sabbagh JJ, Blair LJ, et al: MicroRNA-511 binds to FKBP5 mRNA, which encodes a chaperone protein, and regulates neuronal differentiation. J Biol Chem 291(34):17897–17906, 2016 27334923

5

Epigenetics of Lifestyle and Aging

Kyle J. Rutledge, D.O., Ph.D.
Caroline Gobran, M.D.
Onoriode Edeh, M.D.

The application of epigenetics to mental health is not confined to understanding the development of pathology. Epigenetic signatures and effects are seen in relation to lifestyle measures and the aging process. In particular, the benefits of a healthy diet and exercise and the negative effects of smoking have been found to be mediated in part by epigenetic changes. Rounding out the overview of epigenetics relevant to a psychiatric practitioner, in this chapter we discuss these topics. The review is not exhaustive or in-depth, but rather is meant to provide a glimpse of what has been discovered with respect to these avenues of research, providing important context and a foundation in these branches of study.

Epigenetic Effects of Exercise

Perhaps the most common recommendation to promote health across the life span is to maintain regular physical activity and exercise. Participation in physical exercise is associated with decreased risk of developing a variety of diseases associated with aging. For instance, physical activity has been reported to be a protective and preventive factor against dementia and is associated with lower incidences of cancer, diabetes, and cardiac disease (Bherer et al. 2013). Multiple studies have demonstrated that individuals who participate in regular physical activity—aerobic programs in particular—reduce their cognitive decline with age. Aerobic activity in children is related to improved performance on verbal, perceptual, and arithmetic tasks (Mandolesi et al. 2018). Balance, strength, and resistance training have shown positive effects on cognition. Moreover, physical activity can improve symptoms of depression and anxiety across age groups.

Cognitive benefits from regular physical exercise are coupled with neurological outcomes. Individuals engaging in regular aerobic activity demonstrate decreased loss of both gray and white matter and increased hippocampus size (Bherer et al. 2013). Other studies have shown improved functional connectivity in the brain as well. In animal studies, physical activity has been shown to stimulate angiogenesis and neurogenesis of the hippocampus, increase brain-derived neurotrophic factor (BDNF) (see Chapter 2, "Epigenetic Modulation in Major Depressive Disorder"), and upregulate insulin-like growth factor 1. These effects may provide a partial explanation for the neuroprotective mechanism of physical exercise in humans. At the level of neurotransmitters, physical exercise is tied to increases in serotonin and β-endorphin levels. Together, these molecular and structural neurological effects may explain a large portion of the cognitive, emotional, and behavioral benefits of regular physical exercise.

What is the mechanism through which physical activity exerts these neurological effects? One major player is BDNF, which is essential for neurogenesis, neural development, and synaptic plasticity; notably, physical exercise has been linked to epigenetic changes that can upregulate *BDNF* expression. In contrast, increased methylation of the promoter region of *BDNF*, and subsequent decreased expression, is associated with depression, PTSD, and suicide (Karpova 2014). In a study of rodents, a week of voluntary exercise (access to an exercise wheel) led to decreased methylation of a *Bdnf* promoter region within hippocampal tissue, whereas sedentary rats displayed higher methylation levels within that region (Gomez-Pinilla et al. 2011). Another possible route of physical exercise enhancing *BDNF* expression may be through the function of methyl-CpG-binding protein 2 (MeCP2). MeCP2 can bind to the *BDNF* promoter, suppressing transcription of *BDNF* (see Chapter 3, "Epigenetics in Neurodevelopmental and Neurodegenerative Disorders" for a more thorough review); upon activation, such as through neuronal depolarization, MeCP2 is phosphorylated, detaching from the *BDNF* promoter and opening it up for transcription. In the same rodent study, the authors also found increases in phosphorylated MeCP2, with increased *Bdnf* mRNA levels, indicating upregulated *Bdnf* expression (Gomez-Pinilla et al. 2011). An additional mechanism is that histone 3 acetylation increases with physical activity, which may further contribute to exercise-associated increases in *BDNF* expression in a less specific manner. Therefore, it is likely that a variety of epigenetic effects occur in response to physical activity, leading to neurological effects in part through regulation of *BDNF* expression.

Beyond the direct effects on neural pathways, the benefits of physical exercise may act through mediation of inflammatory pathways. Stressors, whether psychological or physical, can result in release of pro-inflammatory cytokines with downstream systemic inflammatory response, which may mediate the development of mood dysregulation with chronic stress. Long-term physical activity is associated with beneficial effects such as decreased inflammation, which has been tied to increased global methylation patterns (Horsburgh et al. 2015). More specifically, increased physical activity has been associated with DNA hypermethylation of pro-inflammatory tumor necrosis factor genes and DNA hypomethylation of the anti-inflammatory interleukin-10 gene, both linked to decreased inflammation. Therefore, physical activity may yield downstream mental health benefits through modulating inflammatory responses via epigenetic changes.

In addition to changes in DNA methylation, MeCP2 function, and histone acetylation, physical exercise has documented effects on yet another form of epigenetic modification: circulating microRNA (miRNA) levels. Even at low amounts, exercise can affect levels of particular miRNAs (e.g., increase in miR-1 and miR-133a expression) related to improvement in skeletal muscle regeneration, mitochondrial biogenesis, and insulin sensitivity, among other benefits (see Barrón-Cabrera et al. [2019] for a review). Similarly, sedentary behavior is tied to miRNA changes (e.g., decrease in miR-1 and miR-133a expression) related to maladaptive effects such as glucose intolerance. Initiation of physical activity can affect high-density-lipoprotein (HDL)-related miRNA expression in individuals with heart failure, perhaps playing a role in decreasing risk of atherogenesis. In the brain, physical exercise can affect levels of miRNA, with potential protective effects. For example, in mice with traumatic brain injury, miR-21 expression can be altered by exercise, with positive effects on learning and memory that can be reversed when miR-21 expression is artificially adjusted despite exercise (Hu et al. 2015). While research in this area continues to grow, it has become apparent that miRNA provides yet another pathway for exercise to yield benefits for mental health.

Exercise may provide a protective effect against stress-related maladaptive epigenetic effects. In one study, before environmental stress exposure, some rodents were randomized to physical activity, and others were left to remain sedentary (Rodrigues et al. 2015). After stress exposure, authors then evaluated genomewide DNA methylation from brain tissue including cortex, hippocampus, hypothalamus, and periaqueductal gray. Stress exposure led to globally decreased DNA methylation across brain regions in the sedentary, but not the physically active, rodents. In another study, physical exercise was found to reduce expression of miR-124, with subsequent increased glucocorticoid receptor expression in the hippocampus, leading to improved stress resilience (Pan-Vazquez et al. 2015). Therefore, physical exercise may buffer the adverse epigenetic effects of toxic environmental stress.

An additional protective role exercise may play is related to sequelae of chronic alcohol use. One study that examined differences in DNA methylation patterns between binge drinkers and control subjects also examined longitudinal changes to DNA methylation after a 12-month exercise intervention of healthy control subjects (Chen et al. 2018). The authors found an overlap between some loci of exercise-related changes in DNA methylation and the alcohol use comparison; however, the effect was in the opposite direction. Specifically, one of the pathways shown to be affected by epigenetic changes is the reelin pathway, which regulates migration of neurons and maintenance of neural circuits, including the amyloid-β precursor protein (APP) gene. Therefore, although the authors were not examining the effects of an exercise intervention on individuals with alcohol use disorder per se, the results do suggest a potential protective or reversing effect of exercise on some maladaptive methylation changes related to chronic alcohol use, including locations relevant for neurodegeneration.

Interestingly, a greater quantity of exercise is not necessarily better in terms of health outcomes. Individuals who participate in prolonged aerobic exercise, particularly marathon running, may show increased risk for cardiac and inflammatory effects, among others, that are tied to epigenetic mechanisms (see Barrón-Cabrera et al. [2019] for a review). One study examined circulating miRNAs from peripheral blood samples with origins across skeletal and cardiac muscle, as well as inflammatory processes, before, immediately after, and 24 hours after completion of a marathon (Baggish et al. 2014). The authors found all miRNAs to be elevated at the time of race completion, but at different magnitudes, suggesting distinct mechanisms of response rather than a generalized effect to tissues. This altered miRNA expression may be related to observations that marathon running is associated with stress or injury to cardiac and skeletal muscle and increases in systemic inflammation. A direction for future research will be determining whether such effects on increasing systemic inflammation are associated with neurological consequences or downstream effects on cognition or mood.

Diet and Nutrition

"Let food be thy medicine, and medicine be thy food," a quote attributed to Hippocrates more than two millennia ago, underscores how the relationship between nutrition and health has long been appreciated. Indeed, research continues to find new ways in which diet and nutrition play crucial roles in development. More recent work has been incorporating the effects of nutrition and malnutrition at the epigenetic level throughout the course of development.

The **Developmental Origins of Health and Disease (DOHaD)** has become a frequently cited research framework in epigenetic literature that pays particular attention to nutrition and stress in early development. The eponymous international congress continues to update the conceptual model, which primarily focuses on early stages of life with respect to later development of preventable chronic disease, in particular cardiovascular and metabolic disease (Gillman et al. 2007). DOHaD specifically describes research on epigenetics as crucial to expanding our understanding of chronic disease and informing population health efforts to enhance early developmental environments. A large portion of DOHaD research focuses on environmental factors during the fetal stage of development. In terms of pre-/antenatal neurodevelopment and later psychopathology, DOHaD continues to favor broad explanatory models (O'Donnell and Meaney 2017).

Essential to fetal development, the placenta performs a variety of functions that may be affected by its environment. The placenta regulates transportation of nutrients to, and waste from, the fetus, and it regulates the transmission of cortisol. Cortisol passively travels directly across the placenta, but the placenta also produces the enzyme 11β-hydroxysteroid dehydrogenase type 2 (HSD11B2), which inactivates the majority of cortisol passing through before it reaches the fetal bloodstream. Other genes crucial to glucocorticoid function and regulation with respect to the placenta include the glucocorticoid receptor gene *NR3C1* and FK506 binding protein 51 (*FKBP5*; see Chapter 4, "Epigenetics of Childhood Trauma and Resilience," for an overview). Through complex interactions including epigenetic changes, the placenta's gene expression—including expression of glucocorticoid receptors—can be affected by environmental factors

(Clifton et al. 2017). In particular, maternal stress and depression can evoke methylation changes of *HSD11B2*, *NR3C1*, and *FKBP5*, which in turn are associated with greater arousal in newborns and poorer self-regulation, increased lethargy, decreased muscle tone, and other neurobehavioral development changes in the fetus and newborn (Monk et al. 2019).

A significant source of data on downstream effects of malnutrition during fetal development is the Dutch Hunger Winter Famine, which includes a birth cohort from the mid-1940s. Researchers have found that relative to others, including siblings and other family members, individuals undergoing fetal development during the 1944–1945 winter famine in the Netherlands were more likely to develop a variety of diseases, in conjunction with epigenetic marks lasting into late adulthood. The effects were greater for those affected earlier in gestation and were independent of birth weight (see Roseboom [2019] for a review). Neurologically, individuals exposed to the famine in early gestation showed reductions in cortical gray and white matter, in addition to size reductions of the striatum and thalamus. Psychiatrically, studies have shown a wide range of pathology, including increased risk of developing psychotic disorders, mood disorders, addiction, and antisocial personality disorder. Studies examining the epigenetic effects of the famine persisting into late adulthood have shown widespread changes in methylation across multiple genes (Tobi et al. 2009). One such gene is insulin-like growth factor 2 (*IGF2*), which plays a role in neurodevelopment. *IGF2* DNA methylation in postmortem cerebellar samples has been shown to strongly correlate with cerebellar weight (Pidsley et al. 2012). Therefore, early gestational exposure to malnutrition increases risk for a wide range of neurodevelopmental and psychiatric effects, which may be partially explained by persistent epigenetic modifications.

On the other hand, high availability of nutrients has been shown to enhance health outcomes, accompanied by epigenetic changes. A variety of particular bioactive components in foods have been studied, paving the concept of an *epigenetic diet* (see Li et al. [2019] for a review). Fruits and vegetables contain a variety of polyphenols that have antioxidant and anti-inflammatory effects and may affect the machinery of epigenetic modifications. Examples of how these nutrients interact with the epigenome include global effects of inhibition of DNA methyltransferase (DNMT), histone deacetylase (HDAC), and histone acetyltransferase (HAT), as well as regulation of miRNAs. The health benefits of a wide range of plant-based foods in prenatal and early gestational development are thus suggested as a potential protective factor against environmental toxin exposures.

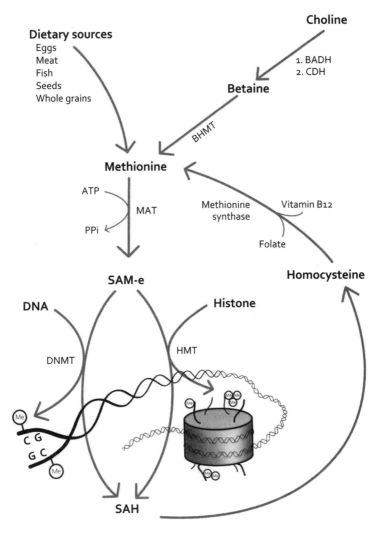

Figure 5–1. Role of SAM-e in DNA and histone methylation.

SAM-e is a methyl group donor for DNA and histone methylation, in the presence of respective methyltransferases. SAM-e is derived from methionine, which is available from dietary sources as well as from biosynthesis pathways involving homocysteine and choline.

ATP=adenosine triphosphate; BADH=betaine aldehyde dehydrogenase; BHMT=betaine-homocysteine methyltransferase; CDH=choline dehydrogenase; DNMT=DNA methyltransferase; HMT=histone methyltransferase; MAT= methionine adenosyltransferase; Me=methyl group, CH_3; PPi=inorganic pyrophosphate; SAH=*s*-adenosylhomocysteine; SAM-e=*s*-adenosylmethionine.
Source. Image by Haley Rutledge, M.S.

Table 5–1.   Epigenetically relevant dietary compounds

Nutrient	Dietary source	Epigenetic effect
Choline	Meat, poultry, fish, eggs, dairy, beans, vegetables, grains	Biosynthesis pathway of SAM, which is crucial for DNA and histone methylation
Diallyl sulfide	Garlic	Increases histone acetylation (HDAC inhibition)
Genistein	Soy	Modulates DNA methylation and DNMT expression and activity
L-Acetylcarnitine	Meat, poultry, fish, dairy	Increases histone acetylation (HDAC inhibition)
Methionine	Meat, poultry, fish, eggs, dairy, beans, nuts, grains	Biosynthesis pathway of SAM, which is crucial for DNA and histone methylation
Resveratrol	Red wine	Involved in histone deacetylation
Sodium butyrate	Biproduct of fiber (legumes, etc.) fermentation in the gut; dairy, cheese	Increases histone acetylation (HDAC inhibition)
Sulforaphane	Broccoli	Increases histone acetylation (HDAC inhibition, DNMT inhibition, miRNA modulation)

See Li et al. (2019) and Tiffon (2018) for more detailed lists.
DNMT = DNA methyltransferase; HDAC = histone deacetylase; miRNA = microRNA; SAM = s-adenosylmethionine.

One of the essential amino acids, methionine, is integral to epigenetic machinery. Through an enzymatic reaction with adenosine triphosphate (ATP), methionine becomes s-adenosylmethionine (SAM or SAM-e), which functions as a methyl group donor (Figure 5–1). SAM-e plays a role in many cellular biochemical pathways, importantly DNA and histone methylation. Therefore, consumption and synthesis of methionine is intrinsic to epigenetic regulation. Food sources rich in methionine include eggs, meat, fish, seeds (such as sesame, hemp, and chia), and some whole grains. Methionine biosynthesis can also involve dietary nutrients including B vitamins (folic acid and B12) and choline from eggs and a variety of meats. Particularly salient examples of epigenetically active nutritional components are included in Table 5–1, and the reader is directed to Li et al. (2019) and Tiffon (2018) for more extensive lists.

Research into the effects of diet on brain and mental health later in life is more limited, but the importance of nutritional elements in epigenetic regulation in older adults has emerged in other branches of medicine such as cancer research (Tiffon 2018). Studying the continued epigenetic effects of diet into adulthood will be a worthwhile future direction of research.

Smoking and Smoking Cessation

Just as substances taken in from the environment may have positive biological effects (nutrients), they may also have negative effects (toxins). Environmental toxins and pollutants have gained attention in applied epigenetic research, predominantly with respect to cancer development. A common example is arsenic, a carcinogen that has been shown to affect DNA methyltransferase expression, with downstream effects on DNA methylation across the epigenome (Rea et al. 2017). Most notably, smoking has emerged as a focus of epigenetic research into the effects of toxin exposure because of its wide prevalence and known significant health consequences. In the field of psychiatry, tobacco use disorder is a common diagnosis across practice settings, whether as a primary complaint or a comorbid condition. As such, a large proportion of patients seeking mental health services are exposed to the toxic effects of smoking, making this avenue of research particularly salient to mental health practitioners.

Smoking has global epigenetic effects, as measured by genomewide changes in DNA methylation. More than 180 specific sites across all autosomes show altered methylation based on smoking status (Zeilinger et al. 2013). The CpG sites isolated by Zeilinger et al. (2013) correspond to promoter regions of genes associated with a variety of cardiovascular, immune, hematological, and reproductive system functions. In a large meta-analysis of genomewide DNA methylation patterns, the authors found differences in methylation patterns related to smoking status across genes tied to the development of cardiovascular disease, pulmonary dysfunction (including chronic obstructive pulmonary disease), osteoporosis, rheumatoid arthritis, and colorectal cancer (Joehanes et al. 2016). Compared with CpG sites relevant for epigenetic age determination (see next section, Aging and the Epigenetic Clock, page 143), Gao et al. (2016) found a significant overlap of sites affected by smoking status and those related to epigenetic age determination, suggesting that a relationship at the level of DNA methylation connects smoking history/status to development of age-related disease (Gao et al. 2016). Further study also determined an overlap between DNA methylation patterns related to smoking and aging-related frailty (Gao et al. 2017). Thus many of the known chronic health effects of smoking have been tied to epigenetic changes, suggesting an etiological role.

The enzyme **monoamine oxidase (MAO)** is moderated by smoking: smokers show increases in expression of the gene, in particular the MAO-B (*MAOB*) isoform (Rendu et al. 2011). MAO has important implications for psychiatry thanks to its role in the metabolism of serotonin, dopamine, and norepinephrine, as well as the therapeutic target of MAO inhibitors. The enzyme is also integral to platelet function and development of cardiovascular disease. Smoking has been found to affect DNA methylation of the gene, with decreases in methylation across CpG sites of *MAOB* and associated increases in MAO expression (Launay et al. 2009).

Exposure to smoking during gestation has been linked to multiple undesirable sequelae, including low birth weight, disease development, pathological neurodevelopment, and infant mortality. A variety of studies of DNA methylation using samples of tissue and blood from mothers, neonates, and placenta have uncovered a possible role of epigenetics in some of these clinical outcomes (Nielsen et al. 2016). Although specific links between these changes to DNA methylation patterns and later development of clinical pathology have yet to be demonstrated, there is an association between the modifications of DNA methylation with smoking and levels of pro-inflammatory protein interleukin-8 as measured in cord blood (van Otterdijk et al. 2017). Furthermore, while there may be some inherited epigenetic effects from preconception smoking exposure, after controlling for smoking status of the mother, father, and grandmother, there emerge distinct DNA methylation patterns corresponding specifically to in utero smoking exposure compared with mothers who had never smoked or had stopped (Joubert et al. 2014).

An encouraging finding from these studies is that the epigenetic changes associated with smoking appear to reverse themselves with smoking cessation. It is possible that early smoking cessation during pregnancy (before 18 weeks' gestation) may undo harmful methylation effects. Wan et al. (2012) examined genomewide methylation of DNA acquired from peripheral blood and found differences in methylation patterns based on whether an individual identified as a current smoker or a past smoker (Wan et al. 2012). Additional dose-dependent patterns emerged with respect to sites showing differential methylation based on cumulative smoke exposure and other patterns linked to time since quitting. In a meta-analysis, the authors found that within 5 years of smoking cessation, the majority of DNA methylation sites affected by smoking showed a return to patterns comparable to those of individuals who never smoked (Joehanes et al. 2016). Other studies have given longer time frames, on the order of decades, before methylation patterns began to match those of individuals who never smoked (Wilson et al. 2017). Regardless, the consistent theme is that of a dose-dependent effect on DNA methylation patterns in smoking cessation, with greater magnitude of methylation change in more intense smokers, as well as greater likelihood of reverting back to nonsmoker status with greater number of years since quitting.

One particular locus of DNA methylation that stands out for its relevant relationship with smoking cessation is that corresponding to the aryl hydrocarbon receptor repressor (*AHRR*) gene, which is involved in cell growth, differentiation, immune function, and response to particular carcinogenic environmental toxins (Zeilinger et al. 2013). This locus has been suggested to have utility as a biomarker for smoking cessation: individuals undergoing smoking cessation therapy demonstrated significant differences in DNA methylation based on whether they were able to successfully quit smoking over 6 months (Philibert et al. 2016). Even individuals who did not quit smoking but decreased their amount of smoking in that time frame showed significant (although more modest) effects in *AHRR* methylation pattern.

The impact of smoking on changes to DNA methylation over the epigenome is relevant in and of itself because of its potential role in the development of smoking-related pathology and chronic disease. The findings are particularly relevant to mental health practitioners given the high prevalence of smoking and tobacco use in our clinical populations. It is likely that those working in mental health fields will regularly encounter patients who have been subjected to prior trauma, environmental stress, or suboptimal inherited patterns—all of which impact the epigenome on their own—plus comorbid smoking with additional epigenetic consequences. It is important to remain vigilant regarding research updates in the field of epigenetics in psychiatry and mental health. Studies of clinical populations must adequately control for smoking within their study design (not just in their statistical models) to account for the robust epigenetic findings associated with smoking.

Aging and the Epigenetic Clock

Research has found applications of epigenetics in the science of aging. Integral to this branch of study is the concept that people, and even tissues within a person, may show changes with age, termed **biological aging**, that are not reliably predicted by chronological age. Therefore, biological markers have been sought to better understand the process of aging and how some individuals appear to progress at rates different from others. Along with the length of telomeres—the end sections of chromosomes that tend to shorten over an individual's life span—DNA methylation levels are related to an individual's age, lifestyle, environment, disease processes, and ultimately, mortality. This phenomenon and measure, the **epigenetic clock**, provides avenues to estimate biological age and opportunities to study factors that may accelerate, decelerate, or even reverse biological aging.

There are methodological variations in how the epigenetic clock is measured or defined, but a common theme is that age can be estimated by a mathematical model incorporating select CpG regions across the genome (see Horvath and Raj [2018] for a thorough review). The regions have been identified through extensive studies and sampling across individuals and tissues. It appears that the particular clusters of CpGs identified do not play a causal role in aging; rather, they are indicators of a global epigenetic process that is related to the process of aging. This measure of biological age can then be compared with chronological age, so within age-matched cohorts, comparisons of various factors can be carried out. This difference between one's epigenetic age (or more precisely, DNA methylation age) and chronological age is referred to as **age acceleration** (when epigenetic age is older than chronological age) or **age deceleration** (when epigenetic age is younger than chronological age). Li et al. (2020) found that only 13% of variation in DNA methylation age is explained by genetic factors, pointing to environmental factors as the predominant cause of variation in DNA methylation age. The authors also demonstrated that early shared environment will affect individuals of the same household similarly, such that cohabitating family members become more similar with respect to DNA methylation age the more time they spend together. This similarity dissipates slowly after separation from the shared environment.

Studies examining epigenetic or DNA methylation age have shown that some variables—such as smoking, obesity, healthy lifestyle, and demographics (education, income, etc.)—relate to aging trajectories and subsequent health status. Furthermore, studies have shown that a variety of pathological conditions may be related to age acceleration, including Down syndrome, Alzheimer's disease, and Parkinson's disease. Epigenetic age is related to measures of frailty of older adults, defined based on ratings of weakness, exhaustion, slow walking, low physical activity, and unintentional weight loss, such that individuals with greater epigenetic age acceleration are more likely to display physical frailty (Gale et al. 2018).

Similarly, individuals with greater epigenetic age acceleration are more likely to perform poorly on measures of lung function, cognition, and grip strength (Marioni et al. 2015b). Finally, epigenetic age has been able to predict all-cause mortality, independent from other genetic, health, or lifestyle factors (Marioni et al. 2015a). Therefore, although the epigenetic markings defining biological age with the epigenetic clock are not necessarily linked to the development of ailments, the patterns may serve as a useful biomarker for age-related health decline.

Additional Topics

Covered briefly here are lifestyle and aging factors associated with epigenetics, and studies continue to explore new directions. Additional research relevant to psychiatric practice have early findings suggesting a role for epigenetic modifications. Some epigenetic effects of mindfulness have emerged, in particular as a treatment for stress and trauma (Bishop et al. 2018). The concept of occupational burnout—emotional exhaustion, cynicism, and reduced accomplishment following prolonged occupational stress—has been a popular topic. Research on burnout is attempting to set a proper definition and identify potential epigenetic biomarkers of the syndrome (Bakusic et al. 2017). Night shift work and irregular work hours, which contribute to shift work disorder and its associated negative health sequelae, are also increasingly studied with respect to epigenetics (White et al. 2019).

Conclusion

The field of epigenetics has countless applications to psychiatry. The science provides a lens to revisit concepts that have been around for millennia, helping us learn more about illness, health, and development. As we work to help our patients, it will be essential to remain familiar with the intersection of epigenetics with psychiatry, as the science brings wonderful opportunities to continue bettering our understanding of mental health and wellness.

KEY POINTS

- Multiple epigenetic effects have been found regarding the health benefits of regular physical exercise. Neurological benefits may come through increases in brain-derived neurotrophic factor (*BDNF*) expression through changes in DNA methylation, methyl-CpG-binding protein 2 (MeCP2) binding, and histone acetylation. Exercise can also reduce systemic inflammation through epigenetic modifications. The epigenetic effects of physical activity appear to be protective, acting as buffers to negative epigenetic consequences of the environment, including stress and alcoholism.

- The Developmental Origins of Health and Disease (DOHaD) framework is frequently referenced in the epigenetics literature. DOHaD primarily focuses on fetal development of chronic disease, including epigenetic effects on the placenta leading to changes in cortisol transmission to the fetus. Dietary nutrients can have effects on epigenetic machinery, with most research focused on nutrient availability during fetal development. Famine may be related to disrupted neurodevelopment, just as availability of nutrients and amino acids may enhance development in part through epigenetic mechanisms.

- Smoking has been tied to robust effects on DNA methylation across the epigenome. Patterns of methylation change are dose dependent—greater exposure yields more pronounced effects compared with nonsmokers—and reversible with smoking cessation after a number of years. The locations of DNA methylation changes with smoking appear relevant for many of the known pathological consequences of smoking, including a variety of cardiovascular, immune, hematological, and reproductive system disorders; pulmonary dysfunction (including chronic obstructive pulmonary disease), osteoporosis, rheumatoid arthritis, and colorectal cancer; and age-related disease and frailty.

- The epigenetic clock posits that methylation patterns across a set of specific CpG sites of the epigenome can provide an estimate of an individual's biological age. This estimate can be compared with chronological age to determine the presence or absence of age acceleration and heightened risk of age-related frailty or pathology versus chronological age—matched peers, potentially giving the measure utility as a biomarker for age-related health decline.

Study Questions

1. By what effect on methyl-CpG-binding protein 2 (MeCP2) may physical exercise increase brain-derived neurotrophic factor (*BDNF*) expression?

    A. Exercise can increase MeCP2 phosphorylation, increasing binding to the *BDNF* promoter.

B. Exercise can increase MeCP2 phosphorylation, decreasing binding to the *BDNF* promoter.
C. Exercise can decrease MeCP2 phosphorylation, increasing binding to the *BDNF* promoter.
D. Exercise can decrease MeCP2 phosphorylation, decreasing binding to the *BDNF* promoter.

Best answer: B

Explanation: MeCP2 is a protein that binds to the *BDNF* promoter region. When bound, MeCP2 will suppress transcription of *BDNF*. When MeCP2 is activated, it undergoes phosphorylation, subsequently releasing from the *BDNF* promoter. With MeCP2 no longer blocking the *BDNF* promoter and inhibiting transcription, *BDNF* expression increases. Exercise has been linked to increased phosphorylation of MeCP2, which decreases binding of the promoter region, ultimately upregulating *BDNF* expression.

2.   The Developmental Origins of Health and Disease (DOHaD) is frequently cited in epigenetics research because it

A. Provides a birth cohort of individuals subjected to famine during fetal development.
B. Emphasizes epigenetics as crucial to understanding the early factors in development of chronic disease.
C. Guides research on familial inheritance patterns of disease.
D. Defines parameters for the epigenetic clock.

Best answer: B

Explanation: DOHaD is a research framework often referenced in clinically relevant epigenetics literature. DOHaD pays particular attention to nutrition and stress in early development, with emphasis on epigenetic mechanisms. A majority of the work is focused on development of preventable chronic disease, with the objective of informing population health efforts and enhancing early developmental environments (answer B). A large portion of DOHaD research focuses on environmental factors during the fetal stage of development rather than familial inheritance patterns (unlike answer C). The Dutch Hunger Winter Famine, which includes a birth cohort that underwent fetal development during the

1944–1945 winter famine of the Netherlands (answer A), and epigenetic effects related to age (answer D) are not specific to DOHaD.

3.   What is the epigenetic role of s-adenosylmethionine (SAM-e)?

A. SAM-e drives methionine biosynthesis, relevant for histone acetylation.
B. SAM-e functions as a methyl group acceptor and is involved in DNA and histone demethylation.
C. SAM-e functions as a methyl group donor and is involved in DNA and histone methylation.
D. SAM-e occupies the promoter region of methyl-CpG-binding protein 2 (MeCP2).

Best answer: C

Explanation: Methionine, which comes either through dietary sources (eggs, meat, fish, seeds, grains) or biosynthesis (eliminating answer A), can produce s-adenosylmethionine (SAM or SAM-e) through an enzymatic reaction with adenosine triphosphate (ATP). SAM-e is crucial to methylation of DNA and histones (answer C), as it is widely used as a methyl group donor (the DNA/histones being the methyl group acceptors of answer B) in these enzymatic reactions. SAM-e does not interact with the promoter region of MeCP2 in a manner that would occupy the promoter region (answer D).

4.   What epigenetic effects have been linked to smoking?

A. Smoking is primarily related to DNA methylation changes in the promoter of the aryl hydrocarbon receptor repressor (AHRR) gene.
B. Smoking leads to permanent changes in DNA methylation.
C. Smoking has negligible effects on DNA methylation, which may be controlled for in statistical models.
D. Smoking has wide-reaching effects on DNA methylation across the epigenome.

Best answer: D

Explanation: Smoking has been linked to changes in DNA methylation patterns across many sites over all autosomes. The locations of these effects have implicated genes relevant for development of pathology across a wide range of body systems (answer D). As the epigenetic effects of smoking are robust, and clinical psychiatric populations carry an elevated risk of comorbid tobacco use disorder, it is not possible to adequately control for the epigenetic effects of smoking through statistical models alone (negating answer C). Many epigenetic effects associated with smoking have been found to be reversible with smoking cessation (negating answer B). Although *AHRR* (answer A) is considered a relevant locus as a potential biomarker for smoking cessation, the epigenetic effects of smoking are much farther-reaching than a single gene.

5. How is biological age determined with the epigenetic clock?

A. Biological age can be estimated by a mathematical model incorporating select CpG regions across the genome.
B. Biological age can be estimated by methylation bands on the ends of chromosomes, which are incorporated into a mathematical model to estimate telomere length.
C. Biological age can be estimated by following methylation patterns that change at a linear rate with age regardless of lifestyle factors such as smoking or obesity.
D. Biological age can be estimated based on the rate of DNA methylation changes, which slow with time.

Best answer: A

Explanation: Biological age (or DNA methylation age) can be estimated by a mathematical model incorporating select CpG regions across the genome (answer A), determined through a variety of prior studies. The identified CpG sites are indicators of a global epigenetic process of aging, which can then be compared with chronological age to determine age acceleration. The methylation patterns of these sites have been found to be related to lifestyle (ruling out answer C), environment, disease processes, and ultimately mortality. Telomere length (answer B) is another, separate, biomarker of age that does not take into account epigenetic modifications occurring over the life span. Estimation of age with the epigenetic clock does not evaluate rate of methylation change (ruling out answer D).

References

Baggish AL, Park J, Min PK, et al: Rapid upregulation and clearance of distinct circulating microRNAs after prolonged aerobic exercise. J Appl Physiol 1985 116(5):522–531, 2014

Bakusic J, Schaufeli W, Claes S, Godderis L: Stress, burnout and depression: a systematic review on DNA methylation mechanisms. J Psychosom Res 92:34–44, 2017 27998510

Barrón-Cabrera E, Ramos-Lopez O, González-Becerra K, et al: Epigenetic modifications as outcomes of exercise interventions related to specific metabolic alterations: a systematic review. Lifestyle Genomics 12(1–6):25–44, 2019 31546245

Bherer L, Erickson KI, Liu-Ambrose T: A review of the effects of physical activity and exercise on cognitive and brain functions in older adults. J Aging Res 2013:657508, 2013 24102028

Bishop JR, Lee AM, Mills LJ, et al: Methylation of FKBP5 and SLC6A4 in relation to treatment response to mindfulness based stress reduction for posttraumatic stress disorder. Front Psychiatry 9:418, 2018 (published correction appears in Front Psychiatry 12:642245, 2021)

Chen J, Hutchison KE, Bryan AD, et al: Opposite epigenetic associations with alcohol use and exercise intervention. Front Psychiatry 9:594, 2018 30498460

Clifton VL, Cuffe J, Moritz KM, et al: Review: The role of multiple placental glucocorticoid receptor isoforms in adapting to the maternal environment and regulating fetal growth. Placenta 54:24–29, 2017 28017357

Gale CR, Marioni RE, Harris SE, et al: DNA methylation and the epigenetic clock in relation to physical frailty in older people: the Lothian Birth Cohort 1936. Clin Epigenetics 10(1):101, 2018 30075802

Gao X, Zhang Y, Breitling LP, Brenner H: Relationship of tobacco smoking and smoking-related DNA methylation with epigenetic age acceleration. Oncotarget 7(30):46878–46889, 2016 27276709

Gao X, Zhang Y, Saum KU, et al: Tobacco smoking and smoking-related DNA methylation are associated with the development of frailty among older adults. Epigenetics 12(2):149–156, 2017 28001461

Gillman MW, Barker D, Bier D, et al: Meeting report on the 3rd International Congress on Developmental Origins of Health and Disease (DOHaD). Pediatr Res 61(5 Pt 1):625–629, 2007 17413866

Gomez-Pinilla F, Zhuang Y, Feng J, et al: Exercise impacts brain-derived neurotrophic factor plasticity by engaging mechanisms of epigenetic regulation. Eur J Neurosci 33(3):383–390, 2011 21198979

Horsburgh S, Robson-Ansley P, Adams R, Smith C: Exercise and inflammation-related epigenetic modifications: focus on DNA methylation. Exerc Immunol Rev 21:26–41, 2015 25826329

Horvath S, Raj K: DNA methylation-based biomarkers and the epigenetic clock theory of ageing. Nat Rev Genet 19(6):371–384, 2018 29643443

Hu T, Zhou FJ, Chang YF, et al: miR21 is associated with the cognitive improvement following voluntary running wheel exercise in TBI mice. J Mol Neurosci 57(1):114–122, 2015 26018937

Joehanes R, Just AC, Marioni RE, et al: Epigenetic signatures of cigarette smoking. Circ Cardiovasc Genet 9(5):436–447, 2016 27651444

Joubert BR, Håberg SE, Bell DA, et al: Maternal smoking and DNA methylation in newborns: in utero effect or epigenetic inheritance? Cancer Epidemiol Biomarkers Prev 23(6):1007–1017, 2014 24740201

Karpova NN: Role of BDNF epigenetics in activity-dependent neuronal plasticity. Neuropharmacology 76(Pt C):709–718, 2014 23587647

Launay JM, Del Pino M, Chironi G, et al: Smoking induces long-lasting effects through a monoamine-oxidase epigenetic regulation. PLoS One 4(11):e7959, 2009 19956754

Li S, Chen M, Li Y, Tollefsbol TO: Prenatal epigenetics diets play protective roles against environmental pollution. Clin Epigenetics 11(1):82, 2019 31097039

Li S, Nguyen TL, Wong EM, et al: Genetic and environmental causes of variation in epigenetic aging across the lifespan. Clin Epigenetics 12(1):158, 2020 33092643

Mandolesi L, Polverino A, Montuori S, et al: Effects of physical exercise on cognitive functioning and wellbeing: biological and psychological benefits. Front Psychol 9:509, 2018 29755380

Marioni RE, Shah S, McRae AF, et al: DNA methylation age of blood predicts all-cause mortality in later life. Genome Biol 16(1):25, 2015a 25633388

Marioni RE, Shah S, McRae AF, et al: The epigenetic clock is correlated with physical and cognitive fitness in the Lothian Birth Cohort 1936. Int J Epidemiol 44(4):1388–1396, 2015b 25617346

Monk C, Lugo-Candelas C, Trumpff C: Prenatal developmental origins of future psychopathology: mechanisms and pathways. Annu Rev Clin Psychol 15:317–344, 2019 30795695

Nielsen CH, Larsen A, Nielsen AL: DNA methylation alterations in response to prenatal exposure of maternal cigarette smoking: a persistent epigenetic impact on health from maternal lifestyle? Arch Toxicol 90(2):231–245, 2016 25480659

O'Donnell KJ, Meaney MJ: Fetal origins of mental health: the developmental origins of health and disease hypothesis. Am J Psychiatry 174(4):319–328, 2017 27838934

Pan-Vazquez A, Rye N, Ameri M, et al: Impact of voluntary exercise and housing conditions on hippocampal glucocorticoid receptor, miR-124 and anxiety. Mol Brain 8:40, 2015 26135882

Philibert R, Hollenbeck N, Andersen E, et al: Reversion of AHRR demethylation is a quantitative biomarker of smoking cessation. Front Psychiatry 7:55, 2016 27092088

Pidsley R, Dempster E, Troakes C, et al: Epigenetic and genetic variation at the IGF2/H19 imprinting control region on 11p15.5 is associated with cerebellum weight. Epigenetics 7(2):155–163, 2012 22395465

Rea M, Eckstein M, Eleazer R, et al: Genome-wide DNA methylation reprogramming in response to inorganic arsenic links inhibition of CTCF binding, DNMT expression and cellular transformation. Sci Rep 7:41474, 2017 28150704

Rendu F, Peoc'h K, Berlin I, et al: Smoking related diseases: the central role of monoamine oxidase. Int J Environ Res Public Health 8(1):136–147, 2011 21318020

Rodrigues GM Jr, Toffoli LV, Manfredo MH, et al: Acute stress affects the global DNA methylation profile in rat brain: modulation by physical exercise. Behav Brain Res 279:123–128, 2015 25449846

Roseboom TJ: Epidemiological evidence for the developmental origins of health and disease: effects of prenatal undernutrition in humans. J Endocrinol 242(1):T135–T144, 2019 31207580

Tiffon C: The impact of nutrition and environmental epigenetics on human health and disease. Int J Mol Sci 19(11):3425, 2018 30388784

Tobi EW, Lumey LH, Talens RP, et al: DNA methylation differences after exposure to prenatal famine are common and timing- and sex-specific. Hum Mol Genet 18(21):4046–4053, 2009 19656776

van Otterdijk SD, Binder AM, Michels KB: Locus-specific DNA methylation in the placenta is associated with levels of pro-inflammatory proteins in cord blood and they are both independently affected by maternal smoking during pregnancy. Epigenetics 12(10):875–885, 2017 28820654

Wan ES, Qiu W, Baccarelli A, et al: Cigarette smoking behaviors and time since quitting are associated with differential DNA methylation across the human genome. Hum Mol Genet 21(13):3073–3082, 2012 22492999

White AJ, Kresovich JK, Xu Z, et al: Shift work, DNA methylation and epigenetic age. Int J Epidemiol 48(5):1536–1544, 2019 30879037

Wilson R, Wahl S, Pfeiffer L, et al: The dynamics of smoking-related disturbed methylation: a two time-point study of methylation change in smokers, non-smokers and former smokers. BMC Genomics 18(1):805, 2017 29047347

Zeilinger S, Kühnel B, Klopp N, et al: Tobacco smoking leads to extensive genome-wide changes in DNA methylation. PLoS One 8(5):e63812, 2013 23691101

Glossary

15q11-q13: Denotation of the area of chromosome 15's long arm, close to the centromere at region 1, covering bands 1–3. This section contains many genes relevant for neurodevelopment, several of which are subject to genomic imprinting, leading to parent-of-origin–specific expression. Genetic errors affecting this region before conception may lead to the development of PWS, Angelman syndrome, or dup15q.

15q11-q13 duplication syndrome (dup15q): A neurodevelopmental disorder that, like Angelman syndrome and PWS, is associated with genes in 15q11-q13. In dup15q, maternal and paternal copies of the chromosome are imprinted, and one copy contains a duplication of the genes in this region, leading to an increased copy number.

adaptation: The genetically programmed development of neural networks based on an experience-dependent maturation process, with subsequent impact on behavior.

age acceleration: The characteristic of a person's epigenetic age (DNA methylation age) being older than their chronological age.

age deceleration: The characteristic of a person's epigenetic age (DNA methylation age) being younger than their chronological age.

allele: One form of two or more variants of the same gene. Alleles are typically heritable and vary from one another in their DNA base sequence, which may result from a difference of a single base or nucleotide, as in a SNP, or deletions or insertions of longer portions of DNA in the gene.

alternative splicing: The condition in which multiple different forms of RNA transcripts may emerge from the same gene. In RNA splicing, some exons may be rearranged or even removed, creating multiple variants or isoforms of mature RNA, which may then be translated into different proteins.

Angelman syndrome: A neurodevelopmental disorder that, like PWS and dup15q, is associated with silencing of genes located in 15q11-q13. In Angelman syndrome, the maternally expressed genes are dysfunctional or absent.

anticipation: The symptoms and features of a genetic condition appearing earlier in life or manifesting more severely as the condition affects subsequent generations. Examples include Huntington's disease and FXS.

anticodon: The three-base-pair sequence complementary to a codon; for example, CAU is the anticodon for AUG.

antiparallel: Oriented in opposite directions.

aryl hydrocarbon receptor repressor (*AHRR*): Gene involved in cell growth, differentiation, immune function, and response to environmental toxins. DNA methylation patterns of this gene appear to correlate with smoking and smoking cessation, as well as PTSD.

autism spectrum disorder (ASD): A neurodevelopmental disorder that emerges in early childhood, with features such as deficient social-emotional reciprocity, abnormal communication, restrictive behaviors, and fixed interests, among others.

autosome: A non-sex chromosome; humans typically carry 22 pairs of autosomes, inheriting one copy from each parent.

base sequence: The order of nucleotide bases of DNA; genetic information.

biallelic expression: The condition in which gene copies (alleles) from both parents are concurrently expressed.

biological aging: Changes with age that are not reliably predicted by chronological age.

bisulfite sequencing: A variant of NGS with an extra step, allowing for location of methylated cytosines in a DNA sample. The addition of sodium bisulfite converts unmethylated cytosine to uracil, while methylated/hydroxymethylated cytosines and other bases remain unchanged. After sequencing, the output shows a sequence of bases that is compared to known standards, revealing the location of unmethylated cytosine bases compared with methylated cytosines.

brain-derived neurotrophic factor (BDNF): A neuronal growth factor widely expressed in the central nervous system that stimulates neuron differentiation, development, plasticity, synaptogenesis, and long-term potentiation. Dysregulated BDNF has been tied to a variety of mental illnesses (e.g., major depressive disorder) in addition to neurodegenerative disorders (e.g., amyotrophic lateral sclerosis, Parkinson's disease, Alzheimer's disease, Huntington's disease) and lack of neuroprotection following cerebrovascular accident.

catechol-*O*-methyltransferase (COMT):   An enzyme (and associated gene, *COMT*) that breaks down catecholamines, including dopamine and norepinephrine. *COMT* is located on 22q11, and polymorphisms are associated with increased risk for development of schizophrenia.

central dogma of molecular biology: Genetic information is passed from DNA to RNA through transcription and RNA to protein through translation. Genetic information is not passed between proteins or backward from protein to DNA.

chromatin: A strand of DNA that has undergone some level of condensation and organization by interactions with proteins (i.e., histones). Chromatin ranges from lightly packed euchromatin to more coiled, condensed heterochromatin. The most condensed form of this structure is referred to as the chromosome.

chromatin remodeling: A dynamic, reversible process by which accessibility of nucleosomes is increased or decreased, with possible influences on rates of gene expression. Mechanisms of chromatin remodeling may include histone modifications (e.g., histone methylation or acetylation) and the effects of other chromatin remodeling complexes.

chromosome: A long, heritable strand of DNA in its most condensed form. Humans typically carry 23 pairs of chromosomes, inheriting one from each parent.

codon: A sequence of three nucleotides, usually abbreviated as the sequence of three bases, that corresponds to a specific amino acid or stop signal during translation. For example, CGA corresponds to arginine; UAG provides a stop signal.

copy number variant (CNV):   In sections of the genome that are duplicated or repeated, an individual may carry a different number of copies than the typical population. Major examples include duplications (an extra copy of one portion of the genome) and deletions (one less copy of one portion of the genome). Sections may be short, as in the case of trinucleotide repeats, or long, encompassing multiple genes.

core promoter: A major segment of the promoter, located just upstream of the transcription start site, that is relevant for staging the preinitiation complex.

CpG island: A sequence of ~1,000 base pairs containing an elevated proportion of cytosine-[phosphate]-guanine (CpG) dinucleotides. CpG islands are mostly unmethylated; however, patterns of CpG island methylation may affect rates of gene expression. About half of CpG islands are within known promoter regions, and the other half (orphan CpG islands) are outside of promoters.

de novo mutation: A mutation, or change to the base sequence of DNA, that is new—that is, not inherited from either parent.

deoxyribonucleic acid (DNA):   A chain of nucleotides comprising deoxyribose, a nitrogen base (guanine [G], adenine [A], cytosine [C], and thymine [T]), and a phosphate group, oriented in such a way that the phosphate group forms the backbone and confers a negative charge (acidic property) to the polynucleotide. The bases are usually oriented to face the medial position when forming a helix.

deoxyribose: A pentose sugar essential for DNA. Differs from ribose in the absence of a hydroxyl group on the carbon atom in the second position.

Developmental Origins of Health and Disease (DOHaD):   A frequently cited research framework and conceptual model in epigenetic literature that pays particular attention to nutrition and stress in early development with respect to later development of preventable chronic disease.

diathesis-stress model: A framework positing the interactive effect of the underlying predisposition to disease (diathesis) with the degree of exposure to stress.

distal promoter: A major segment of the promoter, located farther upstream of the transcription start site than other promoter segments, that includes regulatory sequences such as enhancers, insulators, and silencers.

DNA methyltransferase (DNMT):   An enzyme that facilitates the transition of a methyl group from a methyl donor to a select cytosine base in a sequence of DNA.

downstream: Next in the sequence, relative to the 5′-to-3′ direction.

enrichment analysis: Examples are gene set enrichment analysis (GSEA), network enrichment analysis, or functional enrichment analysis. An application of genomewide DNA analysis in which patterns of over- or underrepresented findings (e.g., DNA methylation) in a sample are compared with previously identified patterns across a network of regions of interest or a gene set. Patterns may be tied to general biological processes, which may then be compared to the study sample.

epigenetic clock: A means of estimating biological age using DNA methylation patterns of specific CpG sites across the epigenome. This complex biomarker, which may help to estimate biological age, suggests factors that may accelerate, decelerate, or even reverse biological aging.

epigenetics: The study of changes in gene products and gene expression without any alteration to the genome base sequence. Epigenetic mechanisms are susceptible to environmental triggers and include DNA methylation and histone modification, which affect a gene's ability to interact with transcriptional machinery, as well as functions of noncoding RNA such as miRNAs, which affect gene expression.

epigenome: The entire compilation of epigenetic marks carried by an individual. The epigenome includes all DNA methylation and histone modification patterns across every chromatin. Some marks of the epigenome are reset before reproduction; others are transmitted to subsequent generations.

epimutation: Errors in epigenetic methylation or imprinting patterns.

euchromatin: A lightly packed, typically more transcriptionally active form of chromatin.

exon: Portion of a gene joined together during RNA splicing into a final mature RNA transcript that may ultimately undergo translation into a protein. Exons are often referred to as coding regions within genes.

expression: 1. The appearance in a phenotype of a characteristic or effect attributed to a particular gene. 2. The process by which genetic information is transmitted from DNA to functional end products including proteins or noncoding RNA.

fetal alcohol spectrum disorder (FASD):   A set of developmental consequences caused by in utero exposure to alcohol.

fetal alcohol syndrome (FAS): A disorder considered to be at the extreme end of FASD, following chronic and heavy alcohol use during gestation.

fetal programming: The effect that environment has in the developing fetus with respect to later pathology, through developmental, genetic, and epigenetic changes.

FK506 binding protein 51 (FKBP5): Co-chaperone of the glucocorticoid receptor complex that inhibits glucocorticoid receptor signaling. FKBP5 hinders the interaction between intracellular glucocorticoid receptor and glucocorticoid, ultimately disrupting the signal pathway by impeding translocation to the nucleus. FKBP5 plays an integral role in the negative feedback loop of the glucocorticoid signal pathway.

fragile X messenger ribonucleoprotein 1 (*FMR1*): Gene encoding FMRP, located on the q arm of the X chromosome. *FMR1* may undergo a trinucleotide expansion of CGG repeats in a region upstream from the coding region, where the number of repeats is associated with decreased expression of FMRP and emergence of symptoms: < 45 repeats is the wild-type variant, 45–200 repeats is considered a premutation and may be associated with symptoms, and > 200 repeats is a full mutation associated with development of FXS.

fragile X messenger ribonucleoprotein (FMRP): An RNA-binding protein understood to interact with many proteins relevant for proper dendrite maturation, synaptic plasticity, and overall neurological development. FMRP is encoded by *FMR1*, which is susceptible to trinucleotide expansions. These expansions occur outside of the coding region and affect the rate of expression, not the structure, of the protein.

fragile X–related elements 1 and 2 (FREE1 and FREE2): Epigenetic boundaries flanking *FMR1*. FREE1 is upstream and FREE2 downstream of the promoter region. Typically, DNA methylation patterns show a notable transition from methylated to nonmethylated at these boundaries, but in FXS, methylation crosses these boundaries, transcending FREE1 and the entirety of the promoter region including the CpGs, transcription start site, CGG repeats, and FREE2.

fragile X syndrome (FXS): A heritable, single-gene disorder associated with *FMR1*.

γ-aminobutyric acid (GABA): The primary neurotransmitter of the brain and spinal cord. GABA plays a role in motor signaling, respiratory rate, proprioception sleep, and anxiety, among others.

gene: A section of DNA that may be expressed. Expression may occur after translation into functional RNA (as in miRNAs and noncoding RNA) or transcription into a protein.

gene set enrichment analysis (GSEA): A method using statistical approaches to identify genes or proteins that are overrepresented and thus may be associated with different phenotypes.

genotype: The particular gene variant (allele) or combination of alleles that an individual carries.

gestational stress: *See* **prenatal stress**.

glucocorticoid receptor: A nuclear receptor that may bind to a glucocorticoid hormone. Upon binding to a glucocorticoid, the glucocorticoid receptor may move into the nucleus and bind to a particular DNA sequence known as the glucocorticoid response element (GRE), then activate or repress transcription of the associated site.

glutamate decarboxylase 1 (GAD1): An enzyme (and associated gene, *GAD1*, located on chromosome 2) that converts glutamate to GABA. Differential expression of *GAD1* has been associated with schizophrenia, among other disorders.

glutamate receptor subunit ε-2 (*GRIN2B*): A subunit of the *N*-methyl-D-aspartate (NMDA) receptor that appears to be susceptible to methylation changes from environmental stressors. Mutations of *GRIN2B* have been associated with a variety of neurodevelopmental and psychiatric disorders.

heterochromatin: A more condensed, typically less transcriptionally active, form of chromatin.

heteroduplex: Hybridization of the RNA and DNA; the genetic recombination of single complementary strands derived from different sources.

histone: A protein essential for chromatin organization. DNA winds around an octamer of core histones (a combination of H2A, H2B, H3, and H4) to form nucleosomes. Linker histones (H1 and H5) further stabilize the nucleosome structure and bind to linker DNA, which joins adjacent nucleosomes.

histone acetyltransferase (HAT):   An enzyme that facilitates the addition of an acetyl group to a histone.

histone deacetylase (HDAC):   An enzyme that facilitates the removal of an acetyl group from a histone.

histone demethylase: An enzyme that facilitates the removal of a methyl group from a histone.

histone methyltransferase (HMT):   An enzyme that facilitates the transition of a methyl group from a methyl donor to a histone.

Huntingtin gene (*HTT*):   A gene located on chromosome 4 that contains a repeating CAG segment within the coding region. CAG coincides with the amino acid glutamine, so the protein product contains a polyglutamine chain that corresponds to the number of CAG repeats within the gene. Having 10–35 repeats is the wild-type variant; higher numbers of repeats, >40, are associated with development of Huntington's disease. With more repeats (longer polyglutamine chains), the protein's three-dimensional conformational structure is altered, although it continues to function. The structural alteration leads to the formation of inclusions within the nucleus and other cell compartments.

Huntington's disease: A neurodevelopmental disorder attributed to a repeating CAG segment within the coding region of a single gene (*HTT*).

hypothalamic-pituitary-adrenal axis (HPA axis):   A hormone-secreting neuroendocrine chain, which includes the hypothalamus, pituitary gland, and adrenal glands, that tightly feeds back on itself and is associated with the body's stress response.

imprinting: The epigenetically controlled preferential expression of one parental allele over the other (i.e., monoallelic expression based on parent-of-origin). The process of imprinting begins in gametogenesis, during which genes may be tagged based on the parent-of-origin. Some genes in some tissues may then be imprinted if only one of the copies is expressed based on these parent-of-origin epigenetic marks. If the maternal gene is imprinted, it is silenced, leaving the gene copy from the father to be expressed (paternally expressed gene). If the paternal gene is imprinted, then the maternal allele is expressed (maternally expressed gene). Imprinting does not refer to the parent-of-origin marks on the genes but rather the entire regulatory process of gene expression based on the parent-of-origin markings.

imprinting control region (ICR): A DNA sequence, found on the genome near imprinted genes, that regulates their expression.

intergenerational transmission: Epigenetic inheritance in gametes formed before trauma exposure.

intergenic: 1. (describing orphan CpG islands) Found between genes; 2. (describing miRNAs) Transcribed independently from neighboring genes.

intragenic: Found within genes (describing orphan CpG islands).

intron: A portion of a gene that is removed from an RNA transcript before translation into a protein. Introns are often referred to as noncoding regions within genes.

intronic: Transcribed along with another gene before being excised during posttranscriptional modification (describing miRNAs).

L-acetylcarnitine (LAC): (aka acetyl-L-carnitine, L-carnitine, carnitine) A compound available through diet and biosynthesis that acts similarly to an HDAC inhibitor. Some research has suggested that LAC has an antidepressant effect through promoting acetylation of histones bound at promoters of genes, increasing expression of the glutamate receptor gene and *BDNF* in neural tissue.

long interspersed element 1 (LINE-1): A repetitive portion of DNA duplicated widely across the genome. In research, methylation of LINE-1 may be used as a proxy measurement for global DNA methylation patterns.

maladaptation: Responses to experiences—commonly toxic environmental stimuli—leading to impacts on neural networks and subsequent behavior patterns that may be dysfunctional across other environments.

messenger RNA (mRNA): An RNA transcript that is translated into a protein.

methyl-CpG-binding domain protein (MBDP): A protein that contains a region able to bind to methylated CpG sites of DNA. After binding to DNA, MBDPs typically attract additional complexes that generally downregulate expression of the associated gene through repressively modifying histones or otherwise increasing chromatin organization. Therefore, MBDPs are essential for the epigenetic regulation of gene expression.

methyl CpG binding protein 2 (MeCP2):   An MBDP that binds to methylated cytosine within CpG islands, affecting regulation of associated genes. The function of MeCP2 is of particular importance for neurodevelopment. Mutations of *MeCP2* (located on the X chromosome) have been implicated in the development of Rett syndrome.

microarray (chip):   A method for genotyping or estimating DNA methylation at multiple sites of a DNA sample at once. A prepared, fragmented DNA sample is washed over a chip containing a library of DNA probes. If the sample contains strands that are complementary to the probes, they bind (hybridize) to those probes. When used for DNA methylation, binding strength at the locations is measured, showing the proportion of methylated cytosines in a given region of interest on the genome. The DNA probes used include many sites of interest on the epigenome, including CpG islands, coding regions, promoters, and enhancers.

microRNA (miRNA):   Small (~18–25 nucleotides), single-stranded, regulatory RNA segments that can silence a gene by posttranscriptionally degrading mRNA or by preventing the attachment of ribosomal subunits, inhibiting translation.

monoallelic expression: The condition in which only one gene copy (allele) is expressed, while the other is silenced. Examples of monoallelic expression include imprinting and X-inactivation.

monoamine oxidase (MAO):   A human enzyme (and *MAO*, the gene encoding it) that breaks down monoamines (in particular, serotonin, dopamine, and norepinephrine). MAO includes two isoforms, encoded by monoamine oxidase A (*MAOA*) and monoamine oxidase B (*MAOB*). Polymorphisms of both isoforms have been associated with development of psychiatric illnesses, and *MAOB* has been found to be susceptible to effects of smoking, with reductions in DNA methylation and subsequent increases in expression. MAOI=monoamine oxidase inhibitor.

mutation: A potentially heritable change to the base sequence of DNA that consists of a substitution, deletion, or insertion of one or more bases.

neuroapoptosis: The functional programmed death of neurons.

next-generation sequencing (NGS):   Also called next-gen sequencing, second-generation sequencing, or massive parallel sequencing. A technique used to determine the sequence of a DNA sample. The sample is broken down into fragments that are fixed to a plate and replicated while being monitored. Data reveal the DNA sequences of the complementary strands synthesized during this process, which are then combined and processed through specialized computational programs, determining the DNA sequence of the entire sample.

nitrogen base: (aka nitrogenous base, base) Nitrogen-containing molecules that are essential components of nucleosides and nucleotides. They include purine bases—guanine (G) or adenine (A)—and pyrimidine bases—cytosine (C), thymine (T), or uracil (U). DNA consists of bases G, A, C, and T; RNA consists of G, A, C, and U.

noncoding RNA: A functional RNA transcript that is not translated into a protein end-product. Noncoding RNAs may serve regulatory functions; examples include miRNAs and *Xist*.

nuclear receptor subfamily 3 group C member 1 (*NR3C1*): Glucocorticoid receptor gene, named based on its classification within steroid receptors.

nucleoside: A molecule comprising a nitrogenous base and a pentose sugar (a nucleotide without a phosphate group). Examples include adenosine, guanosine, thymidine, cytidine, and uridine.

nucleosome: A compact unit of DNA wound around a histone octamer. The appearance of a series of nucleosomes is often compared to beads on a string.

nucleotide: Basic building blocks of the human genome, comprising a nitrogen base, a pentose sugar, and a phosphate group.

orphan CpG island: A section of the genome outside of known gene promoter regions with elevated proportions of CpG dinucleotides. Orphan CpG islands are intragenic (found within genes) or intergenic (found between genes). Although they are outside of promoter regions, methylation of orphan CpG islands may affect regulation of transcriptional activity.

p arm: Conventional name for the shorter of a chromosome's two arms.

penetrance: Of all people with a particular genotype (i.e., carrying a particular gene variant or allele), penetrance is the proportion of those who exhibit the associated phenotype.

pentose sugar: A ring molecule of carbon, hydrogen, and oxygen that may be used in nucleosides and nucleotides. Ribose is used in RNA; deoxyribose is used in DNA.

pharmacoepigenetics: The application of epigenetics to understanding medical treatment response.

phenotype: An observable trait that is an outcome of gene expression and environment. A phenotype may be observable at the cellular level; at developmental, morphological, and functional levels; and at the behavioral level.

pleiotropic: Variants of a single gene locus that produce differences in more than one trait.

polygenic inheritance: A pattern of inheritance in which a trait is passed along by the cumulative effects of multiple genes.

polynucleotide: A chain of nucleotides connected to each other via phosphodiester bonds.

Prader-Willi syndrome (PWS):   A neurodevelopmental disorder that, like Angelman syndrome, is associated with silencing of genes located in 15q11-q13. In PWS, the paternally expressed genes are mutated or absent.

preconception stress: Stressful experiences occurring within a short window of time just before conception.

preinitiation complex: A large group of proteins, including Pol II and multiple transcription factors, that bind to the core promoter, allowing for initiation of transcription of DNA to RNA by Pol II.

pre-mRNA: An initial, precursor mRNA transcript that undergoes posttranscriptional modification, including removal of introns and splicing, before becoming mature mRNA, which may then be translated into a protein.

premutation: A sequence of repeated nucleotides that is longer than in the wild-type allele but may produce no or attenuated disease symptoms. Premutations have a risk of transmitting a full mutation to offspring.

prenatal stress: Stressful experiences occurring after conception but before birth.

primer: Short, single strand of nucleic acid needed to initiate DNA synthesis.

pro-BDNF: A precursor protein to brain-derived neurotrophic factor (BDNF). *BDNF* is a complex gene, with multiple exons and promoters, allowing for multiple different variants (isoforms) of BDNF mRNA transcript. Despite the multiple transcripts being translated into a variety of proteins (pre-pro-BDNF), these products undergo posttranslational cleavage to become the same pro-BDNF protein. Pro-BDNF undergoes further cleavage to yield the functional, mature BDNF protein.

promoter: A DNA sequence along the genome that lies upstream from the transcription start site of a gene. Within this region, proteins including Pol II and transcription factors interact with DNA to carry out translation into RNA. The promoter includes core, distal, and proximal promoter segments.

proximal promoter: A major segment of the promoter located upstream of the core promoter, near the transcription start site, that contains gene regulatory sequences, including CpG islands.

q arm: Conventional name for the longer of a chromosome's two arms.

reelin (RELN): A protein (and associated gene, *RELN*) expressed by GABA neurons key to neurodevelopment (Cajal–Retzius cells), which regulate neuronal migration and synaptic plasticity. Downregulation of reelin, as with disrupted DNA methylation, has been associated with schizophrenia in addition to other neurodevelopmental disorders.

resilience: A buffer for the risk of developing pathological responses to adverse events, containing elements across biological, psychological, and social systems.

Rett syndrome (RTT): A neurodevelopmental disorder caused by mutation of a single gene (methyl CpG binding protein 2 [*MeCP2*]) on the X chromosome.

ribonucleic acid (RNA): A chain of nucleotides comprising ribose, a nitrogen base (guanine [G], adenine [A], cytosine [C], and uracil [U]), and a phosphate group, oriented in such a way that the phosphate group forms the backbone and confers a negative charge (acidic property) to the polynucleotide. The bases are usually oriented to face the medial position when forming a helix.

ribose: A pentose sugar essential for RNA, ribose differs from deoxyribose by the presence of a hydroxyl group on the carbon atom in the second position.

RNA polymerase II (Pol II): A complex of proteins that translates DNA to RNA. Initiation of transcription is facilitated by a group of proteins known as a preinitiation complex. After initiation of transcription, Pol II leaves behind most of the preinitiation complex to continue elongating the transcribed strand of RNA based on the DNA sequence of the gene until reaching a termination signal.

s-adenosylmethionine (SAM or SAM-e):   A compound that acts as a methyl group donor for DNA and histone methylation, among other biochemical pathways. SAM is produced through enzymatic reaction of amino acid methionine with adenosine triphosphate (ATP).

sex chromosome: Chromosomes (designated as X or Y in humans) typically carrying genes that determine biological sex characteristics.

schizophrenia: A psychiatric disorder, conceived in recent years as a neurodevelopmental disorder, diagnosed based on the presence of positive (e.g., hallucinations, delusions) and negative (e.g., prosody of speech, social withdrawal, anhedonia) symptoms.

Simons Foundation Autism Research Initiative (SFARI Gene):   A frequently updated database available to researchers that tracks potential ASD risk genes.

single-nucleotide polymorphism (SNP):   A variation in a single base pair at a specified location on DNA which may be inherited or arise as a result of a mutation. Many SNPs have no effect on the individual (either they occur outside of a coding or regulatory region of a gene or they do not lead to a change in amino acid sequence during translation). Sometimes, SNPs can have effects on phenotype, including drug metabolism or development of pathology.

skewed X-inactivation: An imbalance between maternally versus paternally expressed X chromosomes.

sodium butyrate: (aka butyrate) A compound available from dietary sources or through biosynthesis that acts as an HDAC inhibitor, in addition to further enzymatic effects possibly leading to downstream DNA demethylation. Sodium butyrate may yield antidepressant effects through upregulation of *BDNF* expression.

solute carrier family 6 member 4 (*SLC6A4*):   A gene encoding the serotonin transporter (SERT), also known as 5-hydroxytryptamine transporter (5-HTT), which allows reuptake of serotonin into presynaptic neurons and plays a crucial role in the regulation of emotion, affect, and behavior. Variation in expression of *SLC6A4* has been linked to a variety of mental illnesses including major depressive disorder.

splicing (RNA splicing):   A type of posttranscriptional modification in which portions of precursor RNA (introns) are selectively removed and the remaining portions (exons) are joined together in a process that ultimately yields mature RNA.

stop codon: A sequence of three nucleotides that provide a signal to terminate translation at the end of a gene sequence.

stress: Some force or event that disrupts homeostasis.

stress response: Physiological actions occurring in tandem with protective behaviors necessary to maintain homeostasis.

toxic stress: Prolonged, frequent, or intense adversity.

transcription: The process of converting the base sequence of DNA into RNA.

transcription factor: A protein that regulates the rate of gene expression by binding to DNA. Transcription factors contain DNA binding domains, which allow attachment to particular DNA sequences called response elements. The transcription factors may also form complexes with additional proteins and may act to upregulate or downregulate the rate of transcription of the associated gene.

transgenerational transmission: Epigenetic inheritance in gametes formed after trauma exposure.

translation: The process of converting mRNA into a protein.

trauma: High-intensity stress.

trinucleotide repeat expansion: A DNA mutation in which a series of three nucleotides is duplicated in tandem because of slipped strand mispairing during replication; associated with neurodevelopmental disorders including Huntington's disease and FXS.

tropomyosin receptor kinase B (TrkB):   (aka tyrosine receptor kinase B, tropomycin receptor kinase B, neurotrophic receptor tyrosine kinase 2 [NTRK2]) A receptor bound to the neuron's cell membrane that binds to BDNF extracellularly, leading to a cascade of intracellular effects, ultimately modulating gene expression and influencing neural growth and synaptic plasticity.

upstream: Previous in the sequence, relative to the 5′-to-3′ direction.

variant of uncertain significance (VUS):   A gene form identified in an individual or sample that lacks enough data to indicate whether it is related to the development of a health condition or other clinically relevant outcome.

X-inactivation: In individuals with two X chromosomes, the process by which one X chromosome is markedly condensed, with the effect of significantly downregulating expression of the genes on that chromosome. The process of X-inactivation takes place during embryonic development and involves a combination of both parent-of-origin and random mechanisms. Whichever X chromosome is inactivated is typically maintained over cell replications consistently across life.

X-inactive specific transcript (*Xist*):   A DNA sequence on the X chromosome encoding a functional long noncoding RNA that works to recruit and interact with protein complexes and other repressive epigenetic factors, ultimately leading to chromatin compaction.

X-inactivation escape: Expression of a gene from the otherwise silenced X chromosome despite X-inactivation; evokes a dose difference, which can lead to phenotypic differences and consequences ranging from various disease states to cell death.

Index

Page numbers printed in **boldface** type refer to tables and figures.